Integrating Serious Illness Care into Primary Care Delivery

PROCEEDINGS OF A WORKSHOP

Laurene Graig, Kaitlyn Friedman, and Joe Alper, *Rapporteurs*

Roundtable on Quality Care for People with Serious Illness

Board on Health Care Services

Board on Health Sciences Policy

Health and Medicine Division

The National Academies of
SCIENCES · ENGINEERING · MEDICINE

THE NATIONAL ACADEMIES PRESS
Washington, DC
www.nap.edu

THE NATIONAL ACADEMIES PRESS   500 Fifth Street, NW   Washington, DC 20001

This activity was supported by Purchase Order No. 75N98F20P00009 with the National Institutes of Health's National Institute of Nursing Research and by the American Academy of Hospice and Palliative Medicine, American Geriatrics Society, Anthem, Ascension Health, Association of Professional Chaplains, Association of Rehabilitation Nurses, Blue Cross Blue Shield Association, Blue Cross Blue Shield of Massachusetts, The California State University Shiley Haynes Institute for Palliative Care, Cambia Health Foundation, Cedars-Sinai Health System, Center to Advance Palliative Care, Coalition to Transform Advanced Care, Gordon and Betty Moore Foundation, The Greenwall Foundation, Hospice & Palliative Nurses Association, The John A. Hartford Foundation, Kaiser Permanente, National Coalition for Hospice and Palliative Care, National Hospice and Palliative Care Organization, National Palliative Care Research Center, National Patient Advocate Foundation, The New York Academy of Medicine, Patient-Centered Outcomes Research Institute, Social Work Hospice & Palliative Care Network, Supportive Care Coalition, University of Southern California Leonard D. Schaeffer Center for Health Policy & Economics, and the National Academy of Medicine. Any opinions, findings, conclusions, or recommendations expressed in this publication do not necessarily reflect the views of any organization or agency that provided support for the project.

International Standard Book Number-13: 978-0-309-27433-3
International Standard Book Number-10: 0-309-27433-8
Digital Object Identifier: https://doi.org/10.17226/26411

Additional copies of this publication are available from the National Academies Press, 500 Fifth Street, NW, Keck 360, Washington, DC 20001; (800) 624-6242 or (202) 334-3313; http://www.nap.edu.

Copyright 2022 by the National Academy of Sciences. All rights reserved.

Printed in the United States of America

Suggested citation: National Academies of Sciences, Engineering, and Medicine. 2022. *Integrating serious illness care into primary care delivery: Proceedings of a workshop.* Washington, DC: The National Academies Press. https://doi.org/10.17226/26411.

The National Academies of
SCIENCES · ENGINEERING · MEDICINE

The **National Academy of Sciences** was established in 1863 by an Act of Congress, signed by President Lincoln, as a private, nongovernmental institution to advise the nation on issues related to science and technology. Members are elected by their peers for outstanding contributions to research. Dr. Marcia McNutt is president.

The **National Academy of Engineering** was established in 1964 under the charter of the National Academy of Sciences to bring the practices of engineering to advising the nation. Members are elected by their peers for extraordinary contributions to engineering. Dr. John L. Anderson is president.

The **National Academy of Medicine** (formerly the Institute of Medicine) was established in 1970 under the charter of the National Academy of Sciences to advise the nation on medical and health issues. Members are elected by their peers for distinguished contributions to medicine and health. Dr. Victor J. Dzau is president.

The three Academies work together as the **National Academies of Sciences, Engineering, and Medicine** to provide independent, objective analysis and advice to the nation and conduct other activities to solve complex problems and inform public policy decisions. The National Academies also encourage education and research, recognize outstanding contributions to knowledge, and increase public understanding in matters of science, engineering, and medicine.

Learn more about the National Academies of Sciences, Engineering, and Medicine at **www.nationalacademies.org**.

The National Academies of
SCIENCES · ENGINEERING · MEDICINE

Consensus Study Reports published by the National Academies of Sciences, Engineering, and Medicine document the evidence-based consensus on the study's statement of task by an authoring committee of experts. Reports typically include findings, conclusions, and recommendations based on information gathered by the committee and the committee's deliberations. Each report has been subjected to a rigorous and independent peer-review process and it represents the position of the National Academies on the statement of task.

Proceedings published by the National Academies of Sciences, Engineering, and Medicine chronicle the presentations and discussions at a workshop, symposium, or other event convened by the National Academies. The statements and opinions contained in proceedings are those of the participants and are not endorsed by other participants, the planning committee, or the National Academies.

For information about other products and activities of the National Academies, please visit www.nationalacademies.org/about/whatwedo.

PLANNING COMMITTEE FOR A WORKSHOP ON INTEGRATING SERIOUS ILLNESS CARE INTO PRIMARY CARE DELIVERY[1]

PATRICIA M. DAVIDSON (*Co-Chair*), Vice Chancellor, University of Wollongong, Australia (*as of April 2021*); Dean and Professor, School of Nursing, Johns Hopkins University (*until March 2021*)

PHILLIP RODGERS (*Co-Chair*), Professor, Family Medicine and Internal Medicine, and Co-Director, Clinical Palliative Care Program, University of Michigan School of Medicine (*representing the American Academy of Hospice and Palliative Medicine*)

CLAIRE ANKUDA, Assistant Professor, Geriatrics and Palliative Medicine, Icahn School of Medicine at Mount Sinai

LORI BISHOP, Vice President of Palliative and Advanced Care, National Hospice and Palliative Care Organization

JON BROYLES, Executive Director, Coalition to Transform Advanced Care

KAREN BULLOCK, Professor, John A. Hartford Faculty Scholar, Department of Social Work, North Carolina State University (*representing Social Work Hospice and Palliative Care Network*)

DEBORAH J. COHEN, Professor of Family Medicine, Oregon Health & Science University

CAROLE REDDING FLAMM, Executive Medical Director, Blue Cross Blue Shield Association

ANN GREINER, President and Chief Executive Officer, Primary Care Collaborative

REBECCA A. KIRCH, Executive Vice President, Policy and Programs, National Patient Advocate Foundation

LARS PETERSON, Vice President of Research, American Board of Family Medicine

TAMMIE QUEST, Professor and Chief, Emory Palliative Care Center, Woodruff Health Sciences Center, Emory University

---

[1] The National Academies of Sciences, Engineering, and Medicine's planning committees are solely responsible for organizing the workshop, identifying topics, and choosing speakers. The responsibility for the published Proceedings of a Workshop rests with the workshop rapporteurs and the institution.

Project Staff

LAURENE GRAIG, Director, Roundtable on Quality Care for People with Serious Illness
KAITLYN FRIEDMAN, Associate Program Officer
ANESIA WILKS, Senior Program Assistant
SHARYL NASS, Senior Director, Board on Health Care Services

Consultant

JOE ALPER, Consulting Writer

ROUNDTABLE ON QUALITY CARE FOR PEOPLE WITH SERIOUS ILLNESS[1]

PEGGY MAGUIRE (*Co-Chair*), President and Board Chair, Cambria Health Foundation

JAMES A. TULSKY (*Co-Chair*), Chair, Department of Psychosocial Oncology and Palliative Care, Dana-Farber Cancer Institute; Chief, Division of Palliative Medicine, Brigham and Women's Hospital; Professor of Medicine and Co-Director, Center for Palliative Care, Harvard Medical School

JENNIFER BALLENTINE, Executive Director, The California State University Shiley Haynes Institute for Palliative Care

ROBERT A. BERGAMINI, SSM Health (*representing the Supportive Care Coalition*)

LORI BISHOP, Vice President of Palliative and Advanced Care, National Hospice and Palliative Care Organization

BRYNN BOWMAN, Chief Executive Officer, Center to Advance Palliative Care, Assistant Professor, Brookdale Department of Geriatrics and Palliative Medicine, Icahn School of Medicine at Mount Sinai

KAREN BULLOCK, Professor, John A. Hartford Faculty Scholar, Department of Social Work, North Carolina State University (*representing Social Work Hospice and Palliative Care Network*)

GRACE B. CAMPBELL, Assistant Professor, Department of Acute and Tertiary Care, University of Pittsburgh School of Nursing (*representing the Association of Rehabilitation Nurses*)

JANE CARMODY, Senior Program Officer, The John A. Hartford Foundation

STEVE CLAUSER, Program Director, Improving Healthcare Systems Research Program, Patient-Centered Outcomes Research Institute

SARA DAMIANO, National Director of Palliative Care, Ascension Health

DAVID J. DEBONO, Medical Director, Anthem

---

[1] The National Academies of Sciences, Engineering, and Medicine's forums and roundtables do not issue, review, or approve individual documents. The responsibility for the published Proceedings of a Workshop rests with the workshop rapporteurs and the institution.

CAROLE REDDING FLAMM, Executive Medical Director, Blue Cross Blue Shield Association

ANNA GOSLINE, Senior Director of Strategic Initiatives, BlueCross BlueShield of Massachusetts, Executive Director, Massachusetts Coalition for Serious Illness Care

MICHELLE GROMAN, President and Chief Executive Officer, The Greenwall Foundation

DENISE HESS, Director, Supportive Care, Catholic Health Association of the United States (*representing the Association of Professional Chaplains*)

PAMELA S. HINDS, Executive Director, Department of Nursing Science, Professional Practice & Quality and Research Integrity Officer, Children's National Hospital; Professor of Pediatrics, School of Medicine and Health Sciences, The George Washington University

HAIDEN HUSKAMP, Henry J. Kaiser Professor of Health Care Policy, Harvard Medical School

KIMBERLY SHERELL JOHNSON, Professor of Medicine and Senior Fellow, Center for the Study of Aging and Human Development, Duke University School of Medicine

REBECCA A. KIRCH, Executive Vice President, Policy and Programs, National Patient Advocate Foundation

TOM KOUTSOUMPAS, Co-Founder, Coalition to Transform Advanced Care

SHARI LING, Deputy CMS Chief Medical Officer, Center for Medicare & Medicaid Services

AMY MELNICK, Executive Director, National Coalition for Hospice and Palliative Care

JERI L. MILLER, Chief, Office of End-of-Life and Palliative Care Research, National Institute of Nursing Research, National Institutes of Health

R. SEAN MORRISON, Director, National Palliative Care Research Center, Icahn School of Medicine at Mount Sinai

PHILLIP A. PIZZO, Founding Director, Stanford Distinguished Careers Institute; Former Dean and David and Susan Heckerman Professor of Pediatrics and of Microbiology and Immunology, Stanford University School of Medicine

THOMAS M. PRISELAC, President and Chief Executive Officer, Cedars-Sinai Health System

KITTY PURINGTON, Senior Program Director, National Academy for State Health Policy
JOANNE REIFSNYDER, Executive Vice President, Clinical Operations and Chief Nursing Officer, Genesis Healthcare (*representing the Hospice and Palliative Nurses Association*)
PHILLIP RODGERS, Professor, Family Medicine and Internal Medicine, and Co-Director, Clinical Palliative Care Program, University of Michigan School of Medicine (*representing the American Academy of Hospice and Palliative Medicine*)
JUDITH A. SALERNO, President, The New York Academy of Medicine
LEONARD D. SCHAEFFER, Judge Robert Maclay Widney Chair and Professor, University of Southern California
JOSEPH W. SHEGA, Regional Medical Director, VITAS Hospice Care (*representing the American Geriatrics Society*)
SUSAN ELIZABETH WANG, Regional Chief, Department of Geriatrics & Palliative Medicine, Regional Physician Director, Life Care Planning & Serious Illness Care, and National Lead, Care Management Institute, Palliative Care, Southern California Permanente Medical Group, Kaiser Permanente

Roundtable on Quality Care for People with Serious Illness Staff

LAURENE GRAIG, Director, Roundtable on Quality Care for People with Serious Illness
KAITLYN FRIEDMAN, Associate Program Officer
ANESIA WILKS, Senior Program Assistant
SHARYL NASS, Senior Director, Board on Health Care Services

Reviewers

This Proceedings of a Workshop was reviewed in draft form by individuals chosen for their diverse perspectives and technical expertise. The purpose of this independent review is to provide candid and critical comments that will assist the National Academies of Sciences, Engineering, and Medicine in making each published proceedings as sound as possible and to ensure that it meets the institutional standards for quality, objectivity, evidence, and responsiveness to the charge. The review comments and draft manuscript remain confidential to protect the integrity of the process.

We thank the following individuals for their review of this proceedings:

DEBORAH J. COHEN, Oregon Health & Science University
MARTHA L. TWADDLE, Northwestern Medicine

We also thank staff member **LIDA BENINSON** for reading and providing helpful comments on this manuscript. Although the reviewers listed above provided many constructive comments and suggestions, they were not asked to endorse the content of the proceedings nor did they see the final draft before its release. The review of this proceedings was overseen by **MARK LAZENBY,** University of Connecticut. He was responsible for making certain that an independent examination of this proceedings was carried out in accordance with standards of the National Academies and that all review comments were carefully considered. Responsibility for the final content rests entirely with the rapporteurs and the National Academies.

Acknowledgments

The National Academies of Sciences, Engineering, and Medicine's Roundtable on Quality Care for People with Serious Illness wishes to express its sincere gratitude to the Planning Committee co-chairs Patricia M. Davidson and Phillip Rodgers for their valuable contributions to the development and orchestration of this workshop. The roundtable also wishes to thank all of the members of the planning committee, who collaborated to ensure a workshop complete with informative presentations and rich discussions. Finally, the roundtable wants to thank the speakers and moderators, who generously shared their expertise and their time with workshop participants.

Support from the many annual sponsors of the Roundtable on Quality Care is critical to the roundtable's work. The sponsors include the National Institutes of Health's National Institute of Nursing Research and the American Academy of Hospice and Palliative Medicine, American Geriatrics Society, Anthem, Ascension Health, Association of Professional Chaplains, Association of Rehabilitation Nurses, Blue Cross Blue Shield Association, Blue Cross Blue Shield of Massachusetts, The California State University Shiley Haynes Institute for Palliative Care, Cambia Health Foundation, Cedars-Sinai Health System, Center to Advance Palliative Care, Coalition to Transform Advanced Care, Gordon and Betty Moore Foundation, The Greenwall Foundation, Hospice & Palliative Nurses Association, The John A. Hartford Foundation, Kaiser Permanente, National Coalition for

Hospice and Palliative Care, National Hospice and Palliative Care Organization, National Palliative Care Research Center, National Patient Advocate Foundation, The New York Academy of Medicine, Patient-Centered Outcomes Research Institute, Social Work Hospice & Palliative Care Network, Supportive Care Coalition, University of Southern California Leonard D. Schaeffer Center for Health Policy & Economics, and the National Academy of Medicine.

Contents

ACRONYMS AND ABBREVIATIONS	xix
PROCEEDINGS OF A WORKSHOP	1
INTRODUCTION	1
OPENING REMARKS	3
CREATING A BETTER FUTURE FOR THOSE WITH SERIOUS ILLNESS	7
EXPLORING THE SHARED PRINCIPLES OF SERIOUS ILLNESS CARE AND PRIMARY CARE	8

    Providing Compassionate, Patient-Centered Care for Individuals with Serious Illness, 8
    Normalizing Needs Navigation for All, 9
    Clinical Practice Guidelines for Quality Palliative Care, 12
    The Bridge Between Primary Care and Palliative Care, 15
    Discussion, 17

THE ROLE OF INTERDISCIPLINARY TEAMS IN CARING FOR PEOPLE WITH SERIOUS ILLNESS IN PRIMARY CARE SETTINGS	20

    An Innovative Approach to Caring for High-Risk Patients, 20
    A Social Work Perspective on Interdisciplinary Team-Based Care, 22
    Three Examples of Integrated Care, 24

  Advance Care Planning Shared Decision-Making Tools, 27
  Creating a Primary Care Team to Provide End-of-Life Care, 29
  Discussion, 32
WHAT PEOPLE WITH SERIOUS ILLNESS NEED FROM
PRIMARY CARE: A PATIENT'S PERSPECTIVE   35
POLICY MECHANISMS TO SUPPORT PERSON-CENTERED
CARE FOR PEOPLE WITH SERIOUS ILLNESS IN PRIMARY
CARE SETTINGS   36
  Integrating Serious Illness Care into Primary Care Delivery:
    Focus on Quality, 36
  The Centers for Medicare & Medicaid Services Innovation
    Center: Demonstration Projects to Support
    Comprehensive Care, 40
  Congressional Action to Improve Care for People with
    Serious Illness, 42
  Palliative Care and Serious Disease Management in Primary
    Care, 44
  Discussion, 47
PROMISING INTEGRATED CARE MODELS   50
  Serious Illness Conversations in Federally Qualified Health
    Centers, 50
  The ChenMed Model of Care, 52
  Transforming Urgent Care for Veterans with Serious Illness, 54
  The CARIÑOS Approach: Caring for Persons with Serious
    Illness, 57
  Discussion, 59
CLOSING REMARKS   61
REFERENCES   62

APPENDIX A: Statement of Task   65
APPENDIX B: Workshop Agenda   67

Box, Figures, and Table

BOX

1 Suggestions Made by Individual Workshop Participants to Foster Integration of Serious Illness Care into Primary Care Delivery, 4

FIGURES

1 Results from an unpublished 2019 Patient Advocate Foundation survey of 2,800 patients identifying the top health concerns in limited-resource and underserved populations, 11
2 A stepwise, team-based approach to screening for unmet needs, 14
3 The National Quality Forum measurement framework for palliative care, 39

TABLE

1 The Eight Domains of Palliative Care in the National Consensus Project Clinical Practice Guidelines for Quality Palliative Care Guidelines, 4th Edition, 15

Acronyms and Abbreviations

AAFP	American Academy of Family Physicians
ACP	advance care planning
CMS	Centers for Medicare & Medicaid Services
COPD	chronic obstructive pulmonary disease
COVID-19	coronavirus disease 2019
ECHO	Extension for Community Healthcare Outcomes
EHR	electronic health record
FQHC	federally qualified health center
HEDIS	Healthcare Effectiveness Data and Information Set
HPM CARES	Hospice and Palliative Medicine COVID-19 Action and Resilience Educational Support
MA	Medicare Advantage
NQF	National Quality Forum
PAF	Patient Advocate Foundation
PCP	primary care physician

SHARP	Small, High Acuity/Risk Panel
VA	U.S. Department of Veterans Affairs
VBID	Value Based Insurance Design

Proceedings of a Workshop

INTRODUCTION[1]

Primary care is critical to a robust health care system and improving health equity across diverse populations. An effective primary care system is also vital for improving access to quality care for people with serious illness,[2] which should be informed by the principles and practices of palliative care (Ferrell et al., 2018). Approximately 5 percent of Medicare beneficiaries (2.2 million Americans) are living with serious illness (Kelley and Bollens-Lund, 2017), as are many other non-Medicare eligible individuals, and this number is expected to grow rapidly as the population ages and the prevalence of progressive illness rises. In many communities, particularly urban and rural underserved communities, primary care clinicians are the main workforce caring for people with serious illness, which underscores the need to integrate high quality serious illness care into primary care delivery.

---

[1] The planning committee's role was limited to planning the workshop, and the Proceedings of a Workshop was prepared by the workshop rapporteurs as a factual summary of what occurred at the workshop. Statements, recommendations, and opinions expressed are those of individual presenters and participants, and are not necessarily endorsed or verified by the National Academies of Sciences, Engineering, and Medicine, and they should not be construed as reflecting any group consensus.

[2] "Serious illness" is defined as a condition that carries a high risk of mortality and either impacts a person's daily function or quality of life, or excessively strains their caregivers (Kelly and Bollens-Lund, 2017).

For people of any age, interdisciplinary palliative care teams can relieve symptoms, pain, and stress at any stage of serious illness (CAPC, 2021). Such care is not available to everyone, however. Specialty palliative care, for example, is often only available to those who are in the hospital or enrolled in hospice care. Additionally, it can be difficult for patients to navigate the care they receive from multiple specialists and subspecialists.

Estimates indicate a decline in the available palliative care workforce over the next 20 years while the number of people in need is projected to increase significantly as the population ages (Kamal et al., 2019). One way to address this impending workforce shortage is to improve the ability of primary care clinicians and teams to deliver care informed by palliative care principles and practices to people with serious illness across settings, including home and community (Parikh et al., 2015). These teams are responsible for a significant part of a person's health care, often form strong relationships with patients and their families based on years of trusted care, and are arguably in the ideal position to provide serious illness care precisely because of their relationships with patients whom they may have treated across the lifespan. Furthermore, patients value care continuity and prefer being cared for by providers they know and trust (Gorman, 2016). Developing and enhancing serious illness care delivery by primary care clinicians and practices will require targeted efforts in areas such as education and training of mid-career health professionals, research, credentialing, accreditation, regulation, and payment policy (IOM, 2015).

Increased involvement of primary care clinicians in the care of those with serious illness through end of life is associated with fewer hospitalizations with intensive care unit stays, less care fragmentation and lower overall costs of care (Ankuda et al., 2017). Primary care visits, for example, are associated with reduced hospital and emergency department visits and reduced preventable hospitalizations (Parikh et al., 2015). Integrating palliative care principles and practices into primary care addresses patients' needs in a trusted setting where they receive most of their care and represents a critical element of patient-centered care for people of any age and at any stage of serious illness.

Strengthening the connections between primary care and serious illness care could better serve the needs of the growing number of individuals with serious illnesses. While this may seem to be a natural extension of primary care, the current system focuses mainly on treating acute illnesses and leaves little time for chronic and often progressive conditions (NASEM, 2021; Schmittdiel et al., 2006).

To better understand the challenges and opportunities for integrating serious illness care into primary care settings, the National Academies of Sciences, Engineering, and Medicine's Roundtable on Quality Care for People with Serious Illness hosted a public workshop, Integrating Serious Illness Care into Primary Care Delivery, held virtually via webinars on June 10 and June 17, 2021. The workshop explored the shared principles of primary and serious illness care, the interdisciplinary teams that power both disciplines, the policy issues that can act as barriers to or incentives for integration, and best practices for integrating primary care and serious illness care.

This Proceedings of a Workshop summarizes the presentations and discussions. The speakers, panelists, and participants presented a broad range of views and ideas. Box 1 provides a summary of suggestions for potential actions from individual participants. Appendixes A and B contain the workshop Statement of Task and the workshop agenda, respectively. The speakers' presentations (as PDF and audio files) have been archived online.[3]

OPENING REMARKS

Phillip Rodgers, planning committee co-chair, professor of family medicine and internal medicine, and co-director of the clinical palliative care program at the University of Michigan School of Medicine, opened the workshop by noting the importance of meeting the needs of the growing number of Americans living with serious illness. He pointed out that the current specialty palliative care workforce is insufficient to meet those needs. "All of us deserve the care we need from clinicians we know and trust," said Rodgers. He went on to explain that one of the goals of the workshop was to elevate a conversation about "building a bridge between primary care and serious illness care in order to provide the best care possible for patients and caregivers throughout their journey with serious illness."

---

[3] For additional information, see https://www.nationalacademies.org/event/06-10-2021/integrating-serious-illness-care-into-primary-care-delivery-a-workshop-first-webinar (accessed November 1, 2021) and https://www.nationalacademies.org/event/10-26-2020/integrating-serious-illness-care-into-primary-care-delivery-a-workshop#sectionEventMaterials (accessed November 1, 2021).

BOX 1
Suggestions Made by Individual Workshop Participants to Foster Integration of Serious Illness Care into Primary Care Delivery

Improving Integrated Care Delivery
- Build longitudinal relationships with patients and caregivers to provide a bridge between primary care and palliative care. (Jaén, Stewart, Twaddle)
- Empower relationships between primary care and palliative care and create networks to support primary care physicians (PCPs) and advanced practice providers who are engaged in this care. (Twaddle)
- View patients as human beings, and address them with compassion and empathy. (Roberson)
- Optimize person-centered communication and care coordination across clinicians and care settings by normalizing needs navigation as part of primary care and palliative care clinical guidelines and practice. (Bradshaw, Fingerhood)
- Incorporate social workers into the interdisciplinary care team. (Bullock, Sloan, Twaddle)
- Assess for the caregivers' needs and capacity to be in that role and whether they are at risk for burnout or excessive stress. (Twaddle)
- When developing models of care, consider how they will affect the interdisciplinary team as well as patients. (Sloan)
- Integrate nurses and physician assistants with palliative care expertise into primary care practice and develop relationships with hospice. (Phillips)
- Redefine palliative care as being appropriate at earlier stages of illness rather than as only a near-death option. (Jaén, Phillips, Thompson)
- Enable primary care physicians to have more open conversations that lead to more comprehensive care. (Olex)
- Identify a site champion who can help determine site-specific workflows. (Swiderski)
- Convene champions in primary care, geriatrics, emergency medicine, palliative care, social work, and pharmacy. (Edes)
- Identify roles and responsibilities for every member of the care team. (Patel)
- Standardize needs navigation as part of clinical practice guidelines in order to engage patients from underserved communities and educate patients on the cost of having a serious illness. (Bradshaw)

- Work with the Institute for Healthcare Improvement to integrate "what matters" into practice by training, tracking, and providing feedback on discussing and incorporating "what matters" or patient goals into health record and care plan. (Edes)

Preparing Clinicians for Integrated Care Through Training
- Train clinicians to understand how to coordinate care from a chronic disease perspective. (Olex)
- Increase opportunities to hold virtual grand rounds-type discussions or case-based teaching that will help apply the palliative care guidelines to a particular patient population. (Twaddle)
- Encourage all clinicians to take advantage of resources and learning modules available through the Center to Advance Palliative Care. (Twaddle)
- Provide adequate training to PCPs on symptom management, advance care planning, and other competencies of palliative care as one means of alleviating the need to refer patients to primary care specialists who are in short supply. (Phillips, VandeKieft)
- Train local clergy in remote communities in practices applicable in the palliative care setting. (Bishop)
- Provide coaching and support for clinicians such as during grand rounds and via programmatic-level reminders and refreshers following formal training. (Swiderski)
- Pursue Level 3 American College of Emergency Physicians Geriatric Emergency Department Accreditation. (Edes)

Addressing the Social Determinants of Health
- Elevate social workers to leadership positions to help the interdisciplinary team develop competencies and take actions needed to eliminate disparities and break down the structural barriers that prevent many people of color from accessing palliative and hospice care. (Bullock)
- Support coordinated research, policy, and advocacy to advance the work of social determinants of health screening, standardize needs navigation as a viable intervention, measure the benefits for patients, communities, and programs, and scale these evidence-based approaches to increase quality and expand availability. (Bradshaw)
- Consider culturally appropriate ways of developing and testing interventions that meet the needs of all patients by partnering with community organizations, including Black churches. (Sloan)

continued

BOX 1 Continued

- Develop and test culturally appropriate care models in partnership with people in the community to provide a better understanding of the needs of those being served. (Sloan)
- Develop measures to assess the quality of the cultural, spiritual, and social aspects of care, as well as for caregiver and financial toxicity, to match those for the physical and structural aspects of care. (Kamal)
- Expand the acceptance of palliative care beyond the majority white population by building trust among minority and vulnerable populations. (Barde, Bassano, Bower)
- To transition palliative care from availability to accessibility, champion the workforce, develop quality measures in gap areas, and engage and empower patients and caregivers. (Kamal)
- Within an emergency department, identify seniors at risk and refer them to primary care social workers. (Edes)

Funding Integrated Care Through Payment Reforms
- Advocate for innovative payment models that reward comprehensive, continuous, advanced primary care. (Stewart)
- Use team-based payments to enable primary care practices to be restructured around the interdisciplinary team model and provide equitable, high-quality, patient-centered care. (Jaén, Stewart)
- Expand payment models to include reimbursement for social workers, population managers, chaplains, and other team members who are currently not eligible to be reimbursed for services rendered. (Bishop, Bullock, Phillips)
- Transition away from pay-for-volume to pay-for-value reimbursement. (Barde, Bower, Phillips, Syed, VandeKieft)
- Invest in primary care to enable physicians to have a shared decision-making experience with their patients, incorporate community-integrated health services, and incorporate an improved palliative care into the care delivery model. (Barde, Bower)
- Encourage health plans to provide monthly advance payments for value per member per month to support key activities that occur both during and outside of the traditional office visit, such as referrals, testing, and home-based palliative care. (Barde)
- Encourage payers to create billing codes for interdisciplinary palliative care. (Bower)

CREATING A BETTER FUTURE FOR THOSE WITH SERIOUS ILLNESS

Ada Stewart, president of the American Academy of Family Physicians[4] (AAFP), built on Rodgers's remarks by noting that the U.S. population is aging and increasing numbers of people are living longer with multiple chronic conditions. This underscores the need to ensure sufficient resources to enable primary care physicians (PCPs) and other members of health care teams to deliver high-quality, culturally appropriate palliative and serious illness care to people and communities.

Stewart shared the story of Someji, her patient who has congestive heart failure and chronic obstructive pulmonary disease (COPD), as an example of how principles of serious illness care can be integrated into primary care delivery. Stewart explained that she had many conversations with Someji during their 12-year relationship about what they would do when it came time to decide on end-of-life care. As Someji's condition worsened, he was hospitalized more frequently and seemingly lost interest in talking about his favorite activity, fishing. Eventually, he was admitted to hospice service. Stewart was at his bedside with his family when he died, and she had the opportunity to speak to his wife and children about his wonderful life and his death when they come to see her for their regular medical office visits.

In Stewart's view, the opportunity exists today to create both a better health care system and a better future for individuals like Someji with serious illness. "We need to advocate for innovative payment models that reward comprehensive, continuous, advanced primary care," and help primary care providers meet patients where they are, Stewart explained. Noting that studies have shown how health care systems built on the foundation of primary care improve population health outcomes and advance equity at a lower cost (Erickson et al., 2020; NASEM, 2021; Starfield et al., 2005), she suggested that these systems also produce higher satisfaction among patients and physicians alike. "We need to advocate for those principles, policies, and practices that provide primary care physicians the necessary resources" to accomplish such goals, Stewart emphasized.

Stewart added that addressing issues related to health equity is also a key area of improvement for the health care system. Stewart referenced Reverend Martin Luther King, Jr.'s comment that of all the forms of inequality, injustice in health is the most shocking and inhumane. She emphasized

---

[4] For more information, see https://www.aafp.org/home.html (accessed August 17, 2021).

that "as primary care physicians and family physicians continue to work to improve outcomes and address social determinants of health, it is important to realize the impact that we have in driving conversations around caring for patients with serious illness." She added: "we all have patients like Someji, and we have the ability to meet our patients where they are and provide comprehensive care to them when they need it most."

Stewart concluded by noting that AAFP offers valuable hospice and palliative care resources for its members and the public. She again emphasized the importance of caring for those with serious illness, working together to advocate for and address issues such as innovative payment models, and developing the principles, practices, and policies that will enable PCPs to provide high-quality, culturally appropriate care to their patients in life and at end of life.

EXPLORING THE SHARED PRINCIPLES OF SERIOUS ILLNESS CARE AND PRIMARY CARE

Providing Compassionate, Patient-Centered Care for Individuals with Serious Illness

The first session opened with Shirley Roberson, fellow and member of the board of directors of the Coalition to Transform Advanced Care, who recounted her frustrating and frightening experience when diagnosed with Stage 4 breast cancer. Roberson offered her own experience as an example of how some members of the health care profession have yet to reach the goal of providing compassionate, patient-centered care for individuals with serious illness.

Roberson explained that she had just finished nursing school, did not have health insurance, and was diagnosed after a routine breast cancer screening. Without a PCP and not knowing what to do, she called her local cancer center and spoke with a supportive employee who helped her find a doctor there. Roberson shared that this made her feel like she was finally getting the attention she deserved, rather than being ignored because she did not have insurance.

The cancer center placed Roberson with a group of women who also had breast cancer. Initially opposed to the idea of being in a support group, Roberson realized that "that group is what helped me understand many things." Roberson noticed that the other women were afraid to talk to their doctors because they did not want to anger or annoy them. Roberson came to recognize that most patients with a long-term illness have a pervasive fear that if they complain or say that they are not doing better, they will be punished. "What I learned is that unless you speak up for yourself, unless you defend yourself, unless you are willing to stand up for yourself, nothing is going to take place," she said.

Roberson recounted that one day, a doctor came into the office with a thick folder of papers to discuss the results of a genetic screening test that would help determine her treatment. However, another doctor had already given her the results, and she did not understand why these were different. Roberson noted that each time she tried to ask the doctor about this, he shut her down. Finally, exasperated and angry, she told the doctor to "stop talking and go sit in that blue chair" so that she could explain what she wanted and needed to hear from him. Roberson's oncologist arrived and noticed that she was upset. After a few minutes of talking to Roberson, her oncologist looked through the papers and declared that this was another patient's paperwork.

Roberson explained that by not answering her questions, the first doctor caused her to panic unnecessarily. While she did not disrespect him as a physician, she pointed out that there are times when doctors need to just listen. "The patient needs to feel that you are on his or her side," said Roberson. "You are not just an organ, not just a breast cancer patient, but a human being with human feelings who needs to be addressed with compassion and empathy."

Normalizing Needs Navigation for All

Erin Bradshaw, chief of mission delivery with the Patient Advocate Foundation (PAF), explained that for the past 25 years PAF has delivered effective, compassionate case management primarily to resource-limited people and their caregivers who are coping with complex chronic conditions. PAF's efforts to connect people to safety net programs and other types of assistance are designed to dismantle certain obstacles that they face in gaining access to equitable quality of care. Bradshaw explained, "health equity, diversity, and inclusion are embedded in the core of [PAF's] person-centered agenda." The term "needs navigation" is used to encompass the variety of services that help individuals address unmet health, financial, and social needs while they move through our complex health care system.[5]

---

[5] For more information, see https://www.npaf.org/advocates/volunteer-opportunities/health-needs-navigation (accessed November 3, 2021).

Financial distress, Bradshaw noted, is a reality for many individuals and families dealing with chronic, serious illness (see Figure 1). In an unpublished survey of more than 2,800 patients, many individuals reported that their family's financial viability is a critically important goal of care. With every diagnosis, Bradshaw explained, families face direct cost for medical visits, medications, treatments, indirect costs, such as transportation to care settings, and support needed at home. People also deal with deteriorating health circumstances that interfere with their ability to work, earn an income, or maintain health insurance coverage. Unpaid caregivers often take on additional financial responsibilities and find themselves having to balance caregiving with other work and home responsibilities. Bradshaw explained that PAF case managers hear and address these pressures every day, particularly for populations from low socioeconomic backgrounds, communities of color, and those living in rural regions or medical shortage areas. "This is a very real thing for people and the importance of the untold story behind health inequities," said Bradshaw. "This is an opportunity for us to build upon your roles and help get people what they need and care about at the time of diagnosis."

Bradshaw noted that the services that PAF and other organizations provide often fill in overlooked or inconsistent attempts to improve quality of life outside of the medical setting and that the communities PAF serves have long endured unequal access to care and challenges created by the social determinants of health.[6] Bradshaw also pointed out that the coronavirus disease 2019 (COVID-19) pandemic has drawn much needed public attention to these inequities while intensifying the need for this type of work at the level of individual communities.

Bradshaw emphasized that many people with serious illness have unmet financial and social needs that impact both patient and caregiver well-being. The playbook for primary care, said Bradshaw, should optimize person-centered communication and care coordination across specialists and settings. In fact, she said, now is the time to normalize needs navigation as part of primary care and palliative care practice. Many of PAF's patients that were surveyed reported that the current system-centric health care model is

---

[6] "The social determinants of health are the conditions in the environments where people are born, live, learn, work, play, worship, and age that affect a wide range of health, functioning, and quality-of-life outcomes and risks." For more information, see https://health.gov/healthypeople/objectives-and-data/social-determinants-health (accessed November 10, 2021).

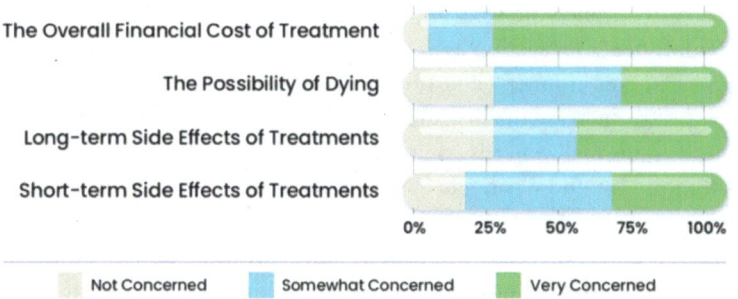

FIGURE 1 Results from an unpublished 2019 Patient Advocate Foundation survey of 2,800 patients identifying the top health concerns in limited-resource and underserved populations.
SOURCE: As presented by Erin Bradshaw, June 10, 2021.

not meeting their needs, as it often forces them to sacrifice basic necessities to pay for recommended treatments. Bradshaw noted that the financial cost of a serious illness is typically unknown to patients or overlooked by health care providers. This lack of knowledge is compounded for patients from underserved communities, who are often not included in all aspects of treatment decision making. Bradshaw suggested that standardizing needs navigation as part of clinical practice guidelines and including all patients in decisions about goals of care would help address patient and caregiver needs.

Bradshaw shared a personal story about her aunt's recent breast cancer diagnosis. She was receiving excellent medical care and successfully navigating treatment, but she faced problems with her employer's medical leave policies. She ultimately lost her job as a result of the complexity and severity of her treatment, when she was just over 1 month shy of qualifying for a disability benefit. This left her without financial assets or resources to support her everyday needs.

Due to her understanding of and experience with the health care system, Bradshaw has been able to fix some of these issues by connecting her aunt with safety net solutions. She also provides family support to help her through the treatment protocol. However, Bradshaw emphasized that not everyone has access to this kind of knowledge or support, which, highlights the importance of standardizing and normalizing needs navigation throughout primary care and palliative care.

Bradshaw concluded by offering strategic steps needed to accomplish that goal. She stressed that coordinated research, policy, and advocacy action is needed to advance the work of social determinants of health screening, standardize needs navigation as a viable intervention, measure the benefits for patients, communities, and programs, and scale these evidence-based approaches to increase quality and expand availability. In short, she said, "we need to normalize needs navigation for all and make sure it is part of the solution. We know patients have access to care, but we want to make sure they have quality [care] and equitable care." In closing, Bradshaw emphasized that these steps will benefit hundreds of thousands of diverse patients and families living in marginalized and underserved communities across the nation.

Clinical Practice Guidelines for Quality Palliative Care

Martha Twaddle, Waud Family Medical Director for palliative medicine and supportive care at Northwestern's North Region and the Northwestern Feinberg School of Medicine opened with reference to the clinical practice guidelines developed by the National Consensus Project for Quality Palliative Care to define and improve palliative care delivery and detail its essential elements. Twaddle explained that the guidelines achieve the following:

- Outline the essential elements of quality palliative care,
- Reflect the multifaceted needs of people and their caregivers as they navigate serious illness and inform decision making,
- Define the structures and process of care and set expectations,
- Provide the framework that enables groups and institutions to set standards and measurements that create a foundation for accountability, and
- Inform policy and payment.

The guidelines were first released in 2001, with a fourth version published in October 2018 (Ferrell et al., 2018).[7] Twaddle noted it included a systematic review of research evidence completed by the RAND Evidence-Based Practice Center and more than 80 national organizations have endorsed the guidelines. The guidelines, said Twaddle, use "serious illness"

---

[7] The guidelines are available in a searchable, online version at http://nchpc.conferencespot.org (accessed August 17, 2021) or to download free of charge at https://www.nationalcoalitionhpc.org/wp-content/uploads/2020/07/NCHPC-NCPGuidelines_4thED_web_FINAL.pdf (accessed August 17, 2021).

to mean "a health condition that carries a high risk of mortality and either negatively impacts a person's daily function or quality of life or excessively strains their caregiver" (Kelley and Bollens-Lund, 2017). This definition, she explained, raises the importance of measuring function, quality of life, and accessibility and understanding how serious illness affects both caregivers and patients. Importantly, this conception of serious illness is not about prognosis, she noted, but rather about the burden of the illness itself and its effects on the patient and caregiver.

The guidelines emphasize that palliative care is, by definition, interdisciplinary. Twaddle noted that when she consults with a patient, she is practicing palliative medicine, which is a medical discipline. Palliative medicine becomes palliative care when she engages with the rest of her team to formulate a holistic, multidimensional perspective for how to best support that person and their family. That interdisciplinary model, said Twaddle, incorporates the six Cs:

1. Comprehensive assessment
2. Care coordination
3. Care transitions
4. Caregiver needs
5. Cultural inclusion
6. Communication

Twaddle shared that she finds the latest iteration of the guidelines to be exciting given the emphasis on supporting both caregiver and patient. "These guidelines assert that one must also assess the needs of the caregiver and the caregiver's capacity to be in that role and whether or not they are at risk for burnout or excessive stress, because it does take a village," she said. Twaddle pointed out that as Bradshaw noted in her comments, the formal caregiver cannot always do it all, so access to additional caregivers and navigators is needed. The latest guidelines also stress sensitivity to culture and ethnicity and inviting the patient and family to identify their preferred modes of communication. For example, Twaddle explained that the first question she asks patients focuses on the amount of information they find helpful. This is important because not everyone wants to know everything. Next, she asks the critical question of who the patient wants to have with them when they receive information that could be life changing or redirecting.

Twaddle noted that there is some blurring of roles when the interdisciplinary team works well, as team members can screen for unmet needs outside of their expertise. For example, Twaddle, can conduct an initial screen for unmet social needs, but a social worker performs the in-depth assessment. Similarly, Twaddle can screen for unmet spiritual needs, but the team's spiritual care provider would conduct the in-depth assessment (see Figure 2). Twaddle emphasized that no team can practice palliative care without a social worker given the huge role that social needs and social determinants play. She also noted that in community-based palliative care, the active piece of spiritual care often comes from the community.

Twaddle explained that the clinical practice guidelines are constructed to reflect the domains of palliative care (see Table 1). She pointed out that each guideline provides a general description of and criteria for the specific domain. Domain 1 contains the broadest guideline in that it details team composition, how to provide care, and the transitions of care.

Twaddle noted that sections also detail the clinical implications of the guidelines, essential palliative care skills that clinicians need to carry out the guideline, an overview of the research supporting the guideline for each domain, and real-life, nationwide examples that illustrate how communities, services, or groups of people found ways to meet the needs of the seriously ill in their communities. These examples, said Twaddle, are meant to be inspirational—and to provide a reminder that it is impossible to have care teams of professionals with every expertise needed by patients with serious illness.

Twaddle concluded by noting that clinicians need to think broadly about other care team members. She pointed out that

> [t]here are some essential folks, depending on our population, that I feel we need to have closely knit within our practice model, but we may be collaborating with community-based spiritual care and we may be collaborating with care managers from certain agencies to meet the very diverse needs of our patient population.

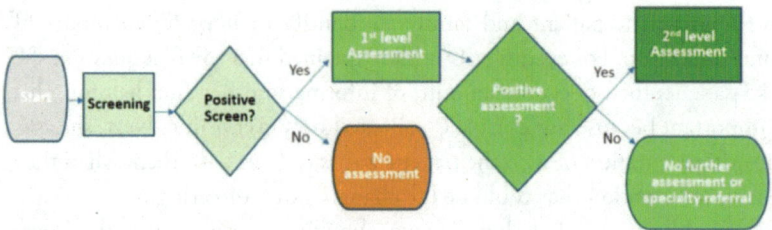

FIGURE 2 A stepwise, team-based approach to screening for unmet needs.
SOURCE: As presented by Martha Twaddle, June 10, 2021.

TABLE 1 The Eight Domains of Palliative Care in the National Consensus Project Clinical Practice Guidelines for Quality Palliative Care Guidelines, 4th Edition

Domain	Aspect of Care
Domain 1	Structure and Processes of Care
Domain 2	Physical Aspects of Care
Domain 3	Psychological and Psychiatric Aspects of Care
Domain 4	Social Aspects of Care
Domain 5	Spiritual, Religious, and Existential Aspects of Care
Domain 6	Cultural Aspects of Care
Domain 7	Care of the Patient Nearing the End of Life
Domain 8	Ethical and Legal Aspects of Care

SOURCES: As presented by Martha Twaddle, June 10, 2021; National Consensus Project for Quality Palliative Care. Clinical Practice Guidelines for Quality Palliative Care, 4th edition. Richmond, VA: National Coalition for Hospice and Palliative Care; 2018. https://www.nationalcoalitionhpc.org/ncp.

The Bridge Between Primary Care and Palliative Care

Carlos Roberto Jaén, the Dr. and Mrs. James L. Holly Distinguished Chair, professor and chair of family and community medicine at the Joe R. and Teresa Lozano Long School of Medicine at the University of Texas Health San Antonio, opened by noting that primary care and palliative care clinicians share a focus on a biopsychosocial model[8] of clinical practice. He identified the pillars of biopsychosocial clinical practice as

- Self-awareness,
- Active cultivation of trust,
- An emotional style characterized by empathic curiosity,
- Self-calibration as a way to reduce bias,
- Educating the emotions[9] to assist with diagnosis and forming therapeutic relationships,
- Using informed intuition, and
- Communicating clinical evidence to support dialogue (Borrell-Carrió et al., 2004).

---

[8] For more information on the biopsychosocial model, see Engel (1977).
[9] For more information on emotional education, see Epstein (1999).

Referring back to Roberson's experience with her own care, Jaén pointed out that her story was a good example of the lack of cultivation of patient trust by clinicians.

Jaén illustrated the pillars of biopsychosocial care with quotes from two family medicine practitioners. The first doctor said,

> I believe that family doctors will always be generalist trained, relationship centered, and community oriented. We are generalists not by virtue of what we do or know, but in the way we ask questions and construct solutions in response to the suffering of those who sit before us. We trust the looping arc of conversation, one that leads to a deeper understanding and sense of belonging. We know the value of patience, reassurance, and gentle guidance, of talk when impatient action would soothe only the doctor's insecurities. (Loxterkamp, 2019)

The second doctor said: "what could be of greater comfort and safety to patients and their families than to have a trustworthy physician as counselor and advocate during the vicissitudes of a critical illness, chronic progressive disability, and dying? That and a loving family are the best protections that I could wish for myself or anyone who wants to avoid the horror of dying" (Stephens, 1990).

Reiterating that palliative care physicians alone cannot meet the needs of everyone who could benefit, Jaén noted how important it is to activate, affirm, and support primary care's participation in serious illness care. He noted that the shared principles of primary care[10]—notably person- and family-centered, continuous, comprehensive and equitable, team-based and collaborative, coordinated and integrated, accessible, and high-value care—are similar to the principles that Twaddle articulated for palliative care.

Jaén pointed out that the National Academies consensus study report *Implementing High-Quality Primary Care* provides guidance on relevant policy issues and a revised definition of primary care, which articulates high-quality primary care as "the provision of whole-person, integrated, accessible, and equitable health care by interprofessional teams that are accountable for addressing the majority of an individual's health and wellness needs across settings and through sustained relationship with patients, families, and communities" (NASEM, 2021, p. 4). This definition, he said, places responsibility on the interprofessional team, promotes agency, and

---

[10] For more information, see https://journals.stfm.org/familymedicine/2019/february/epperly-2018-0288 (accessed August 17, 2021).

emphasizes the role of communities. The report also lists five objectives for achieving high-quality primary care:

1. Payment—pay for primary care teams to care for people, not doctors to deliver services.
2. Access—ensure that high-quality primary care is available to every individual and family in every community.
3. Workforce—train primary care teams where people live and work.
4. Digital Health—design information technology that serves the patient, family, and interprofessional care team.
5. Accountability—ensure that high-quality primary care is implemented in the United States.

Jaén observed that health care reform in the United States has, for too long, focused on how primary care will help save the nation money. The primary care study, however, argues that high-quality primary care is a common good similar to public education, and cost savings should not be considered to be the major driver. The report makes the case for creating a central office of primary care in the U.S. Department of Health and Human Services to ensure the resources exist to support quality primary care, palliative care, and coordination between the two disciplines (NASEM, 2021).

In closing, Jaén echoed Rodgers's statement that primary care can serve as a bridge to palliative care by providing collaborative, optimal care. "However, some patients, particularly in my community, are blocked from getting to the bridge because they do not have access, while some get to the bridge too late," said Jaén. Many PCPs, he added, welcome the opportunity to accompany their patients during a difficult journey. Jaén shared that based on his personal experience, such care provides clinicians with a wonderful opportunity to experience gratitude.

Discussion

To open the discussion session, moderator Claire Ankuda, assistant professor of geriatrics and palliative medicine at the Icahn School of Medicine at Mount Sinai, asked the panelists to share their perspectives on the common ground between primary care and palliative care. Twaddle responded that for her, the two fields are integrated and interwoven and the model of approach is the same in that the idea of relationship-based care is focused on the person and the family. Stewart agreed that the two disciplines are both about relationships and having the necessary tools to adequately serve patients and family members: the patient and family are at the center of care for both. Twaddle also emphasized that it is precisely the relationships with the patient and family that enable primary care to provide palliative care to those facing serious illness.

Jaén echoed both Twaddle and Stewart, noting that the role of primary care is in building longitudinal relationships. The synergy that comes from working together with palliative care colleagues also provides the necessary transition. He added that there are many people with conditions that might not traditionally be thought of as serious illness. These people, however would also benefit from the whole-person care and services that integrated serious illness and primary care can provide.

Bradshaw commented that the medical care that people with serious illness receive through primary and palliative care is extremely important. She stressed the importance of acknowledging the impact of serious illness on a person's identity and recognizing their nonmedical needs. A holistic and community-based approach can help support a patient's unmet needs, which may be less readily apparent than their medical needs.

When asked if the priority for integrating primary care and palliative care was to have more collaboration or to train primary care clinicians to integrate palliative care principles into their practice, Jaén, Twaddle, and Stewart all replied that both were priorities. Given the insufficient numbers of palliative care specialists to provide care for every person in need, Twaddle cited the importance of empowering relationships between the two disciplines and creating networks to support PCPs and advanced practice providers who are engaged in this care. Stewart added that the only way to ensure that everyone has the opportunity to access high quality, culturally appropriate, and equitable care is to provide every health care team with the necessary tools to accomplish that goal.

Twaddle added that such care is not always continuous. She noted some patients with whom she uses her palliative care skills might not come in for years at a time but return needing holistic, multidimensional support. "It is about using the essential elements and applying [them] to the right population," she said.

Ankuda then asked Twaddle about strategies for disseminating the guidelines and related trainings. Twaddle replied that training opportunities are increasing within palliative care. For example, several institutions now offer online master's programs. She noted the networks of palliative care experts that clinicians can call upon for guidance and that the COVID-19 pandemic has given rise to widespread acceptance of virtual training and online coaching. Twaddle shared that she envisioned increasing opportunities to hold virtual grand-rounds-type discussions or case-based teaching that will help apply the guidelines to a particular population and that the next iteration of the guidelines will work on closer alignment with primary care.

An audience member asked Roberson for her thoughts on how to enable and support patients to have the courage she demonstrated when speaking to clinicians. Roberson replied that the first thing is the importance of having a strong desire to stay alive, which should translate into the ability to ask questions and tell the doctor when some piece of information is unclear. Twaddle remarked that one of the competencies in palliative care concerns communication that centers on the patient. When she talks to a patient about shared decision making, she emphasizes that while she has the disciplinary knowledge, the patient has the lived experience. The combination creates a powerful opportunity to make better decisions. In fact, she invites and encourages her patients to rebut her recommendations if these are contrary to what they want.

Roberson observed that most physicians do not engage in shared decision making. In her experience, most doctors will even remind a patient how little time they have to spend or to explain things at the patient's level. Stewart encourages her patients to pose questions through written lists or via patient portals. She acknowledged that despite plenty of resources to help physicians learn how to better communicate and partner with their patients, the profession needs to do more to make sure they are aware of and actually use those resources.

Jaén noted that an additional part of good communications is coordinating with the entire team. If there is a discrepancy, it is the responsibility of the clinicians to find out the source and make sure they are all on the same page. In fact, he believes that one role for the primary care team is to be the patient's advocate and ally and work with them throughout their journey. Sometimes, that will involve disagreeing with a specialist about a course of action, though the responsibility to resolve such issues remains with the PCP rather than the patient.

Regarding Roberson's comment about physicians not having enough time to be responsive and listen to patients, Twaddle said it is important for primary care to push back and better manage its schedules to reflect the time demands that come with properly treating patients with serious illness. In Stewart's opinion, the key will be restructuring primary care practices to better reflect the interdisciplinary team model, which will depend on changing the way payment for services is focused. Stewart and Jaén share the perspective that payment reform is essential for health care teams to provide equitable, high-quality patient-centered care.

Concerning provider education, Twaddle pointed to the resources and learning modules available through the Center to Advance Palliative Care. She also noted that additional resources such as VitalTalk[11] can provide assistance with learning to communicate more effectively with patients, though such skills training is best practiced in a forum that can provide coaching. Stewart added that the AAFP has resources available on hospice and palliative medicine.

THE ROLE OF INTERDISCIPLINARY TEAMS IN CARING FOR PEOPLE WITH SERIOUS ILLNESS IN PRIMARY CARE SETTINGS

An Innovative Approach to Caring for High-Risk Patients

Marianne Logan Fingerhood, track coordinator for the adult/gerontological nurse practitioner program, program director for the Supporting Nursing Advanced Practice Transitions (SNAPT) fellowship, and assistant professor at the Johns Hopkins School of Nursing, opened the second workshop session. Fingerhood explained that she and her colleagues reviewed the care they were providing for people with serious illness and identified care integration as a significant problem. Poorly integrated care led to increases in hospitalizations, visits to PCPs, and increased costs of care. Fingerhood said that a number of social factors may put someone in the high-risk category, including where they live, access to healthy food, and how much support they have from family members. These patients, she explained, have multiple comorbidities, including COPD, heart failure, and diabetes, and many have had multiple hospital admissions. "Our aim is to be able to care for patients in their homes and in the community rather than through multiple hospitalizations," she said.

In order to provide such care, Fingerhood and her colleagues developed the Small, High Acuity/Risk Panel (SHARP) program to improve care coordination and enhance accountability to their patients and their families. Fingerhood explained that the SHARP program is made up of

---

[11] Additional information is available at https://www.vitaltalk.org (accessed August 17, 2021).

teams led by nurse practitioners, who work closely with PCPs and registered nurses who are responsible for triage and follow-up. The teams include a pharmacist—a key member given the number of people requiring multiple medications—and a social worker who helps with mental health concerns, addresses disparities, and connects patients with needed nonmedical supports. The SHARP program teams coordinates care with a variety of subspecialists including:

- A home care group whose staff assists with care coordination, particularly after hospital discharge;
- A physical therapy group that provides outpatient care, including in the home;
- An occupation therapist that works with people and their families to help them attain the ability to care for themselves in their own homes; and
- An internal palliative care and hospice group.

Fingerhood explained that the SHARP program primarily identifies patients that would benefit from extra care through reports of multiple hospitalizations over a 6-month period, frequent office visits, and/or Healthcare Effectiveness Data and Information Set (HEDIS) measures for individuals that imply that the care offered was not meeting goals specific to their illnesses. In addition, she and her colleagues explore whether end-of-life planning is appropriate given an individual's condition.

These patients, said Fingerhood, already have an established relationship with their PCP, who has usually determined that the individual patient needs improved care. Fingerhood pointed out that as a PCP, she typically has 15–30 minutes to care for each of her patients. This time allows her to make an initial plan, but a SHARP team can meet with a patient for an hour to identify any gaps in their care that may be addressed by subspecialists. Being able to collaborate with PCPs and redistribute some of their responsibilities to subspecialists has been incredibly important for ensuring patients have continuity of care, said Fingerhood.

A significant component of coordinating care involves the SHARP team's communication with the person, their family members, and the subspecialists—all with the goal of ensuring the patient is at the center. The SHARP team also focuses on building trust, demonstrating respect, providing emotional care, and meeting the critical social needs of both the patient and family that are often neglected. As a result, said Fingerhood, satisfaction for patients and their families has been "amazing." She concluded by noting that, in addition to respecting and supporting patients and their families, interprofessional teamwork has been integral to caring for these high-risk patients and adequately conducting long-term planning to ensure their needs are met.

A Social Work Perspective on Interdisciplinary Team-Based Care

Karen Bullock, professor and head of the School of Social Work at North Carolina State University, explained that long before COVID-19, it was well established that social workers were essential members of health care teams for individuals with serious illness. Bullock pointed out that the United States has more than 600,000 professional social workers (NASW, n.d.) and that social work is a value-based profession whose members function in accordance with the values, ethics, and standards of the National Association of Social Workers Code of Ethics.[12] Cultural competence, a core component of that code, requires knowledge, awareness, humility, skills, and observable practice behaviors that are central to evaluating effective practice.

Bullock emphasized that high-quality integrated primary care successfully merges behavioral health and medical health services. "When patients are seeking interventions for a physical health condition, they are often also dealing with psychosocial needs and these may accompany and be intertwined with the health condition that they are presenting with," said Bullock. "We, as social workers, must assess for this intersectionality," she added.

Bullock explained that advocacy is one of the cornerstones of the social work profession in that it champions the rights of individuals and communities with the goal of achieving equity. In that regard, distributive justice is an important concept to consider in interdisciplinary and integrated care for people with serious illness, because it helps reimagine the notion of counterbalancing wealth and power in the allocation of health care resources and services. Bullock added that this can create the means for eliminating disparities.

Bullock pointed out that professionally trained social workers focus on the comprehensive factors that affect an individual's health and wellness. For social workers, serious illness care includes treatment planning, coordination of care, administration of services, and a host of other skills

---

[12] Additional information is available at https://www.socialworkers.org/About/Ethics/Code-of-Ethics/Code-of-Ethics-English.

to address the needs of relieving suffering for people with serious illnesses. Psychological, emotional, social, and spiritual support, and behavioral approaches to pain management and other psychosocial services, are within the social worker's domain as a means of assisting and supporting patients and families. All of this activity, said Bullock, occurs in the context of a relationship that considers what the patient was experiencing before entering the care system.

Bullock said she appreciated Roberson's comments about the lack of shared decision making she experienced in her care and noted that she often hears similar accounts from her patients or in her research. In fact, she had a similar experience when her mother was diagnosed with metastatic lung cancer and entered a system of care that was not aligned with her values, resulting in care that was not goal concordant.

Bullock stressed that social workers can be at the core of serious illness care by providing services either at hospice centers or in the person's home. Hospice-based social workers in particular receive specialized training and education to provide services in community-based care settings and to follow-up with patients who need intensive medical care during hospital visits. Palliative care social workers may also conduct home visits to assist patients and families in establishing effective home-based care and can act as advocates with medical providers. Bullock noted the importance of starting with understanding what the patient's experience with serious illness has been before they entered the care system. Social workers, added Bullock, receive specialized, competency-based training through the Association of Palliative and Hospice Social Workers to conduct such assessments and work in the hospice and palliative care setting.[13]

Bullock noted that social workers have a critical role as members of primary care teams for those living with serious illness. In addition to conducting assessments of need, they can assist with treatment planning, reevaluation, care coordination, ensuring goal-concordant care, and addressing structural racism. Social workers can play a key role in helping the team develop the competencies and take actions to eliminate disparities and break down the structural barriers that prevent many people of color from accessing palliative and hospice care.

Social workers are often viewed as the "quiet members" of the care team who help the team work together to provide the best care that meets the

---

[13] Additional information on this training and certification program is available at https://aphsw-c.org (accessed August 17, 2021).

needs of patients and their families, according to Bullock. Providing culturally based and congruent care can sometimes be challenging, and social workers are well equipped to help teams think about the ways they assess these challenges. Moreover, social workers are the team members who will be familiar with the resources available in both the primary care and community settings to provide equitable, culturally congruent care.

In closing, Bullock emphasized that the COVID-19 pandemic has shed light on the essential role of social workers in providing care for those with serious illness. "Our perspective of distributive justice is one that can be useful as a guiding framework for identifying structural barriers to not only hospice and palliative care, but [also] serious illness care in general for many Black and brown people who continue to be at risk for greater morbidity and mortality. As team members, social workers are equipped to help you create opportunities and access to address greater health equity and serious illness care," Bullock concluded.

Three Examples of Integrated Care

Gregg VandeKieft, medical director of the palliative practice group at the Providence Institute for Human Caring and a palliative physician and clinical ethicist with Providence St. Peter Hospital, shared his experiences with three projects that are integrating serious illness care into primary care. The first project, the Washington Rural Palliative Care Initiative,[14] began in 2017 and is a public-private partnership of more than 24 organizations sponsored by the state department of health's Office of Rural Health and funded by a number of private, state, and federal sources and in-kind contributions. The project builds on work by Stratis Health,[15] a quality improvement organization based in Minnesota whose efforts developed palliative care services in 23 rural Minnesota communities and additional locations in rural North Dakota and Wisconsin.[16]

VandeKieft explained that the objectives of the Washington project are to assist rural health systems and communities in their efforts to integrate palliative care in multiple settings. The project aims to better serve people

---

[14] For more information, see https://waportal.org/partners/home/washington-rural-palliative-care-initiative (accessed August 17, 2021).

[15] For more information, see https://stratishealth.org (accessed August 17, 2021).

[16] For more information, see https://stratishealth.org/initiative/rural-community-based-palliative-care (accessed September 9, 2021).

with serious illness in rural communities, decrease transfers to distant urban tertiary services, move upstream to serve people with serious illness earlier, and develop care models for sustainable services. The project began in 7 communities and has since added 10 more. The locations include a waterfront, a sea-going fishery, timber, rangeland, farmland, orchards, and retirement communities. At the time of the workshop, 14 of the 17 communities remained active in the project, while the others were more passively involved as a result of reduced staffing and administrative resources.

VandeKieft said that each local team has a local leader, 12 of whom are nurses. The teams are based in critical access hospitals, federally qualified health centers (FQHCs), primary care practices, and home health programs, and at least one is an innovative collaboration of clinical and community-based volunteers. Participants also cross the spectrum of disciplines with nurses being the most common, then physicians, social workers, nurse practitioners, chaplains, pharmacists, physician assistants, dieticians, paramedics, and nursing assistants.

The model for creating these teams started with community engagement and education efforts led by the Office of Rural Health, whose staff conducted in-person site visits to all seven of the initial communities. They were conducting site visits for the second 10 communities when the COVID-19 pandemic struck, forcing the visits to become virtual. These site visits, explained VandeKieft, are intended to build relationships in the community and educate both clinicians and community members about serious illness care. They include an in-depth assessment of community assets and a gap analysis to determine the resources needed to build bridges between palliative care, primary care, and the community.

Starting in mid-2018, VandeKieft and his colleagues began case consultations in which the community-based primary care teams virtually bring cases to a specialized palliative care team. He noted that the program does not yet perform direct consultations with patients. At the end of a session, the project's nurse coordinator puts together a detailed summary of discussion points and recommendations and sends it to the community-based providers as guidance. For the first seven sites, these consults occurred twice per month; currently they are once per month. He noted that at least three of the local teams have expanded their operation to create a blended in-person, onsite model that includes direct-to-patient telemedicine visits by a physician accompanied by simultaneous onsite visits from social workers, nurses, and chaplains to perform full-spectrum palliative care consults.

Vandekieft explained that detailed data on outcomes are still pending. However, a comparison of the patient emergency department use, hospitalizations, length of hospital stay, and rate of referrals to hospice for the 6 months prior to and after enrollment found a dramatic reduction in the first three factors. The evaluators also found that the participants felt better integrated into their community after enrolling in the program.

VandeKieft also discussed Project Extension for Community Healthcare Outcomes Hospice and Palliative Medicine COVID-19 Action and Resilience Educational Support (ECHO HPM CARES). It is a collaborative effort that includes Four Seasons Compassion for Life, Providence Health System, Cambia Health Foundation, and the ECHO Institute at the University of New Mexico. He explained that the original Project ECHO[17] was developed to provide specialized hepatology services for individuals with hepatitis C in rural communities in New Mexico who had trouble getting to Albuquerque for advanced subspecialty care. VandeKieft noted that the original project produced distinct improvements in outcomes and a greater appreciation among specialists in the city for what care is like in rural communities.

Project ECHO has almost 400 hubs for more than 100 diseases in 44 countries,[18] and internal registration data show that ECHO HPM CARES has participants from 34 states. The project's meetings alternate between palliative care and hospice cohorts. VandeKieft noted that 852 attendees had participated in these sessions at the time of this workshop, 5 percent of whom joined for more than 10 sessions and 144 who attended both a hospice and a palliative care session. He added that Four Seasons Compassion for Life in North Carolina started Project ECHO HPM and invited his team at Providence to join the project. However, in response to the pandemic the program switched from general outreach to focusing on COVID-19-related outreach. Preliminary unpublished survey results indicate that 95 percent of participants felt they were better able to work in an interdisciplinary team and 92 percent felt more motivated to communicate with other team members and discuss how teamwork can contribute to continuous and reliable patient care.

VandeKieft ended with a description of the Providence Medical Group's Oregon Region initiative to enhance primary palliative care skills

---

[17] For more information, see https://hsc.unm.edu/echo/about-us (accessed November 3, 2021).

[18] For more information, see https://hsc.unm.edu/echo/partner-portal/data-marketplace/interactive-dashboards (accessed September 9, 2021).

across the state's 50 primary care clinics and 150 subspecialty clinics.[19] Every clinical person in each primary care clinic will receive foundational VitalTalk training. Intermediate-level training will include 4 weeks of specialized training over 1 year, and those who receive training at this level will serve as trainers for the foundational course. The goal is to have at least one person from each clinic participate in the University of Washington's graduate certificate program in palliative care and 48 people across the state become palliative care specialists for both the inpatient and outpatient settings. Internal quality measures show that, at the time of the workshop, the program had produced a nearly 7 percent increase in the number of primary care patients who completed advance directives and a 15 percent increase in a specific type of goals-of-care documentation.

In closing, VandeKieft summarized that each of the three projects has a shared focus to engage and train members of the interdisciplinary team and a shared commitment to accomplish more in the primary care setting before having to turn to specialty palliative care.

Advance Care Planning Shared Decision-Making Tools

Danetta Sloan, assistant scientist at the Johns Hopkins Bloomberg School of Public Health, opened by noting that social workers in hospice are the team members who most often have conversations with patients and families about advance care planning (ACP). They have the challenge of balancing patients' values with the needs of the institution to have an advance directive completed quickly and saved in the patient's medical record.

Sloan described her work on a study funded by the Agency for Healthcare Research and Quality[20] evaluating the effectiveness and implementation of interventions for integrating palliative care into ambulatory care for adults with serious, life-threatening illness and their caregivers. Sloan and her colleagues evaluated interventions addressing patient identification, patient and caregiver education, shared decision-making tools, clinician education, and models of care. They explored five specific areas:

1. How can we identify those patients who could benefit from palliative care in ambulatory care settings?

---

[19] For more information, see https://oregon.providence.org/our-services/p/providence-medical-group (accessed September 10, 2021).

[20] For more information, see https://www.ahrq.gov (accessed August 17, 2021).

2. What educational resources are available for patients and caregivers in ambulatory care about palliative care?
3. What palliative care decision-making tools are available for clinicians, patients, and caregivers in ambulatory care?
4. What educational resources are available for non-palliative care clinicians about palliative care in ambulatory settings?
5. What are the models for integrating palliative care into ambulatory settings?

Sloane noted that in terms of the third question, all the shared decision-making tools identified by the study team were designed to assist ACP or goals-of-care conversations. While they concluded that such tools may improve patient satisfaction with communications, the strength of evidence was low in part because the sample sizes were small. The review also found that these tools may increase the documentation of advance directives, though the strength of evidence was similarly low. "We really could not draw any conclusions about the effect of shared decision-making tools on caregiver satisfaction or patient symptoms of depression," said Sloan, adding that "no studies addressed other critical outcomes."

Sloane pointed out that the study found that patients and caregivers preferred ACP discussions grounded in patient and caregiver experiences of illness rather than general conversations about the end of life and the study revealed that the timing should be individualized to the specific situation of the patient and caregiver. In social work, this is called "meeting the patients where they are," said Sloan. The results of the study also demonstrated that clinicians preferred ACP shared decision-making tools that were time-efficient and included structured scripts.

Sloan explained that her team assessed the available decision-making tools by meeting with key informants, including professionals, patients, caregivers, and interdisciplinary team members. This qualitative evidence indicated that the tools should be grounded in patient and caregiver experiences of illness. The qualitative evidence emphasized that interventions should be time-efficient, specific, and succinct. However, Sloan noted that effectiveness studies that included comprehensive interventions conducted by additional staff outside of the routine workflow directly challenged integrating these tools into ambulatory care. Lastly, the qualitative evidence from patients and caregivers also emphasized the importance of considering the timing of interventions as well as patient and caregiver preferences.

Sloan stressed that it is important when developing models of care to think about how they will affect the interdisciplinary team as well as the patients. She noted that none of the studies her team was able to abstract assessed equity, addressed disparities, or mentioned diversity. She said, that studies need to explore culturally appropriate ways of developing and testing interventions that meet the needs of all patients. One way to do that is by partnering with community organizations, particularly Black churches. For example, 93 percent of the 937 church members Sloan surveyed said they wanted more information on end of life and ACP (Hendricks Sloan et al., 2016).

In closing, Sloan urged workshop attendees to develop and test any care models in partnership with people in the community to ensure they are responsive to people's needs. She also called for developing culturally appropriate models that integrate training for the interdisciplinary teams serving those communities.

Creating a Primary Care Team to Provide End-of-Life Care

Russell Phillips, director of the Center for Primary Care at Harvard Medical School, opened by talking about his own experiences as the division chief for general medicine, where he had the opportunity to create interventions within the institution's hospital-based practice. One such intervention involved inserting a palliative care specialist into primary care practices, with the surprising result that the specialist's services were rarely used. Phillips said main reason was that the PCPs were reluctant to assign end-of-life decision making to others. "In addition, we did not surround them with a system that supported their work," Phillips said.

Phillips listed the seven principles of chronic or severe illness care, which are aligned with those developed by the Patient-Centered Primary Care Collaborative[21]:

1. Patient, family, and community centered;
2. Continuous and relationship based;
3. Comprehensive and equitable care for all, from first contact to end of life;
4. Team-based, collaborative, and inclusive of social workers, nurses, and clergy;

---

[21] For more information, see https://www.pcpcc.org (accessed August 17, 2021).

5. Coordinated and integrated-with open channels of communication;
6. Accessible at all times, day or night; and
7. High value that extends time for patients and prevents unwanted services, especially at the end of life.

The Collaborative Care Model is one that he and his colleagues have worked on over the years, and Phillips noted that the strong evidence base showing how important it can be for patients with depression (Gilbody et al., 2006; Katon et al., 2010; Unützer et al., 2002). This model not only reduces the cost of care but improves symptoms of depression and can prevent mortality due to suicide (Gallo et al., 2013). The patient-centered care team is a critical component. Phillips explained that applying the model to palliative care would require a team with PCP, an advanced practice nurse or physician assistant with expertise in end-of-life care, a population health manager to track patients, and a medical assistant to help identify symptoms and screen patients for entry into what might be a registry for following patients.

Phillips noted a variety of ways to identify patients with serious illness. One approach is to ask physicians the surprise question: "Would you be surprised if your patient passed away in the next year?" Though this metric has been shown to be an accurate risk factor for mortality, it should be used in conjunction with other screening techniques (White et al., 2017). Excellent prognostic indexes also exist, said Phillips, that could be applied to the electronic health record (EHR) or billing data. In Phillips's view, it should be possible to create registries for patients with severe, chronic illness that population health managers could follow.

Once a patient is identified, Phillips noted that palliative care clinicians could talk with PCPs or advance practice providers about the person's care preferences, health care proxies, or preferences for site of care at death (i.e., home versus hospital). In addition, clinicians could discuss the advantages and disadvantages of hospice care and gauge patients' interest level. Medical assistants could then monitor symptoms over time and identify poorly controlled symptoms that might include depression and substance use, explained Phillips. This would trigger necessary interventions such as diagnostic tests, treatments, and referral to a palliative care specialist. Finally, there would be continuous and regular visits with the PCP, advanced practice nurse, or physician assistant that would continue when the patient entered hospice. He said that he likes to be the physician on record when someone enters hospice and that he visits patients at home when they are in hospice or no longer mobile.

Phillips identified a number of barriers and facilitators to applying the Collaborative Care Model to palliative care. One of the largest barriers is payment, given that population health managers and other team functions are not covered under most plans. Phillips noted that one way to address this barrier would be to transition to value-based prospective payment (also known as capitation[22]) with supplements for palliative care, supportive care, and care management services that include all team members and virtual care. Quality metrics, severity adjustment, and incentives to serve as the hospice care physician of record would also help, said Phillips.

Expertise is key when it comes to end-of-life care, and programs such as Project ECHO can provide that training. Phillips's institution has developed learning collaboratives. In addition, it should be possible to develop nurse specialist roles within practices. In Phillips's experience, patients want care from their PCP at the end of life. Moreover, most PCPs want to provide that care and believe that end-of-life care is vital for both patients and their families.

In addition to training clinicians on symptom management, ACP, and other palliative care competencies, several additional reforms are needed to facilitate integrated palliative specialty care. For example, patients need to be informed about the benefits of palliative care and hospice. The delivery system itself would benefit from finding ways to integrate nurses and physician assistants with palliative care expertise into primary care practice. Phillips shared that he typically works with different hospices, which requires him to simultaneously care for a patient at the end of life and create referral guidelines for palliative care specialists.

In closing, Phillips pointed out that payment policy reform is needed to create a way to adequately pay for care of patients with serious illness, preferably using capitation. Other policy options include efforts to reinforce primary care competencies among all health care providers. Finally, palliative care needs to be redefined as appropriate at earlier stages of illness rather than as a near-death option, concluded Phillips.

---

[22] Capitation payments are a fixed amount of money paid per patient per unit of time paid in advance. For more information, see https://www.acponline.org/about-acp/about-internal-medicine/career-paths/residency-career-counseling/guidance/understanding-capitation (accessed November 3, 2021).

Discussion

Moderator Lori Bishop, vice president of palliative and advanced care at the National Hospice and Palliative Care Organization, opened by noting that the Center for Medicare & Medicaid Innovation has committed to implementing a palliative care model demonstration. Along with the National Coalition for Hospice and Palliative Care, her organization has been pushing for a model that is in close collaboration with primary care. "We feel that relationship is a sacred one and we want to know how we can complement each other," she said.

When asked about reimbursement for the SHARP program, Fingerhood explained that the program was initially funded by a grant from Maryland Medicare and was supplemented by capitated payments. Fingerhood noted that the SHARP program is realizing some cost savings that it can use. VandeKieft stated that the Oregon project was made possible by the high percentage of value-based contracts in the Oregon marketplace and that it would have never worked in a traditional fee-for-service environment. "The payers were incentivized to try and determine how we can best meet the patient's" pre-acute care needs he said. "We often talk about post-acute care, but they are really focusing from a population health mindset on pre-acute care." He acknowledged that the model would not work as well in other markets simply because the payment structure would not work, and until the nation moves to more value-based contracting, the spread of this type of model will be constrained.

Phillips explained that his hospital does a great deal of value-based contracting, but the money does not flow to primary care. Rather, it comes into the organization and is distributed according to a fee-for-service approach. He pointed out that primary care only receives 5 percent of the nation's total medical spending, which is much less than it needs to provide all the essential services (Bailit et al., 2017; Koller and Khullar, 2017). "Certainly, when we think about adding new services such as integrated palliative care, we need to find ways to increase that payment to closer to 10 to 15 percent of the total medical spend, and we are working toward that in Massachusetts," said Phillips (Phillips and Bazemore, 2010; Koller, 2017).

Bullock commented that most people who work as a part of a team acknowledge that social work adds value, yet it is challenging for those services to be reimbursed in the same way as other clinical services. That issue, she said, contributes to the lack of available social work services on teams, which then affects care. The social work profession, she added, is working hard to develop mechanisms, such as competency-based certification, to ensure reimbursement for the services that social workers provide.

Bishop noted that chaplains have the same problem as social workers even though chaplaincy is a core service, and Sloan added that chaplains and clergy are now being included in evidence-based research to demonstrate their value as part of the interdisciplinary care team. VandeKieft said a huge gap remains between the acute care setting and hospice in terms of spiritual care support. In his experience, philanthropy provides support for chaplaincy services in community-based palliative care. He explained that when his clinic first opened, it had foundation funding for a chaplain in the clinic setting, but when the grant ran out he could not secure additional funding. The chaplain now talks to the clinic team virtually and works with the embedded social worker. VandeKieft said that many teams end up deferring to the patient's own clergy member. VandeKieft pointed out that while this approach has tremendous value, there is a gap between the services provided by a clinically trained chaplain[23] and one's own clergy member.

Bishop commented that when she worked in a rural community that had a very distinct religious base for the majority of the population, end-of-life discussions were difficult because they were considered unacceptable. Sloan wondered if it might be possible to set up programs to train local clergy in remote communities in practices applicable in the palliative care setting. Bullock noted that many clinicians ask her about inequity and she tells them that bringing in untrained clergy who are not of the same faith as the patient can be a form of inequity, because the patient's needs are not being adequately met.

In terms of inequity in palliative care and hospice services, Sloan said that hospice organizations need to pay attention to the diversity of their teams and ensure that team members are comfortable about meeting the needs of patients who come from a different racial, ethnic, religious, or other cultural community. Sloan and Bullock noted that some hospice providers are concerned about going into neighborhoods or even homes they

---

[23] In the United States, all chaplains undergo clinical training, known as clinical pastoral education. "A clinically trained chaplain is a professionally trained clergy member who helps navigate the health care system. They can support patients and staff with a variety of belief systems, faiths, and cultures." For more information, see https://spiritualhealth.emory.edu/_includes/documents/sections/research/training-healthcare-chaplains.pdf (accessed November 3, 2021).

perceive as dangerous. Bullock noted insufficient training to help people feel comfortable going into homes to provide care.

When asked about the role of mental and behavioral health in serious illness care, Bullock said that many patients who are receiving care for a physical condition will have a psychosocial or behavioral health issue such as anxiety or depression. Social workers, she noted, are trained to assess whether a given patient living with serious illness needs behavioral health care. VandeKieft added that in the patient-centered medical home, behavioral health care is a crucial part of holistic primary care long end-of-life or serious illness care. "The more we can design primary care systems that incorporate mental and behavioral health care from the get-go, the more it can be integrated throughout the full spectrum of care," said VandeKieft.

Fingerhood commented that most PCPs recognize the need for mental and behavioral health care, but access to those health care professionals can be difficult in many organizations. Phillips agreed with that assessment and noted that even referring patients to behavioral health services in the community is challenging because either the resources do not exist or the providers do not take insurance. Insurance coverage is definitely a barrier, added Bullock, to which Bishop observed that it is hard to get whole-person care when whole-person insurance coverage is not within reach.

Bishop raised the issue of workforce shortages, which are forcing primary care and palliative care to compete for workers, and asked how the two disciplines might work together more collaboratively to expand the sense of team to meet workforce needs. VandeKieft replied that the Oregon model he discussed recognized this problem and decided on an augmentation approach that trains people in primary care to have a higher level of palliative care skills. This leaves referrals to palliative care specialists for the most complex cases, and it also is more efficient from a population health mindset for meeting people's needs. "In a value-based contracting model, that is going to be much more prevalent than if we remain in our piecemeal fee-for-service model that so many people are still stuck in," he said. Phillips suggested that the eConsult model that enables virtual consults with specialists could help. He added however, that the model is not covered under fee-for-service models either, even though it has been shown to reduce costs (Anderson et al., 2018; Gleason et al., 2017; Liddy et al., 2016; Vimalananda et al., 2015). In Phillips's view, this is another reason to move toward value-based capitated payment; for palliative care, those specialists are often not available. Making sure that we are using them as efficiently as possible is really critical, and eConsults offer a way forward," he concluded.

WHAT PEOPLE WITH SERIOUS ILLNESS NEED FROM PRIMARY CARE: A PATIENT'S PERSPECTIVE

To provide another perspective of someone living with serious illness, the second webinar opened with a presentation by Mike Olex, a person who has multiple sclerosis. A former medical physicist, Olex is now a volunteer with PAF and active advocate in the multiple sclerosis and disability communities. Olex opened by recounting being diagnosed with multiple sclerosis 16 years earlier. He noted that while he realized that the diagnosis would change his life, he did not foresee it as becoming all encompassing. His condition has forced him to give up his profession and activities that he loved, such as hockey. He now relies on a wheelchair for mobility.

Olex explained that while his PCP and a host of other specialists have provided care over the years, getting that care has not always been easy. Olex shared that he is responsible for his own care coordination, which is challenging. "I am having to coordinate, manage, and be the expert on my own care, which I do not mind, but at the same time, I do not necessarily know who to reach out to even coming from the perspective of being in the health care system for well over a decade professionally." He added that the majority of people with serious illness face this same problem. Olex shared that he often reaches out to a friend or colleague in the advocacy community for referrals. In one instance, that led him to a specialist who understood the difference between caring for a seriously ill patient in his early forties, with the need to get his illness under control for the next 30–40 years, versus someone in their sixties or seventies.

While he is now on medication that has stabilized his condition, Olex also wants to manage his illness holistically through weight loss, stretching, and other activities that can help him so that he does not have to rely exclusively on medication for the next several decades. One of Olex's biggest concerns was his loss of balance and coordination, yet this was never addressed by his PCP or his neurologist, who, in Olex's view, seemed to have the attitude that this was the way his life would be. But for Olex, a former hockey player, good coordination and balance was a major part of who he was and represented something that primary care should have addressed and probably would have if he had had a good, ongoing relationship with his PCP.

Olex noted that because he is no longer physically active, he now has type 2 diabetes and takes medication to treat it. He has lost weight and his diabetes is now well controlled, but he worries about the long-term impact of being on that medication. Olex emphasized that what he needs from his primary care team is advice on what he can do for his diet. However, Olex's experience has been that clinicians prescribe medications rather than having a discussion about diet or giving a referral to a dietician.

Olex explained that when he worked as a medical physicist at a cancer center, the care team would get together on a regular basis to develop multi-step care plans and coordinate care among the many specialists involved in caring for a patient. "That is not something we have when it comes to comprehensive care for someone with multiple sclerosis or anything like that," said Olex. In his experience, patients are pigeonholed into one of four main types—relapsing, remitting, progressing, or acquiring clinically isolated syndrome—and those designations do not translate into plans that will help patients live their best lives over the long term.

Olex recalled that when he was no longer able to walk without assistance, he had to coordinate getting a walker, a power scooter, a wheelchair, and eventually a power wheelchair. No playbook existed, he said, that could have helped him with each of those tasks. He explained that even though the majority of people with multiple sclerosis will not end up in a power wheelchair, it should not be that difficult to have guidance available for those who do. The same should be true for medications, he added. He is now on his ninth disease modifying therapy; if he had not been his own advocate, he probably would still be on earlier, less effective medications.

In closing, what Olex would like to see from primary care is not necessarily that his provider becomes his friend, but that they help him understand how to manage his illness and coordinate his care from a chronic disease perspective. Above all, he would like the relationship he does have with PCP to be one in which he is able to talk frankly, ask as many questions as he likes, and not have to rely on finding a specialist.

POLICY MECHANISMS TO SUPPORT PERSON-CENTERED CARE FOR PEOPLE WITH SERIOUS ILLNESS IN PRIMARY CARE SETTINGS

Integrating Serious Illness Care into Primary Care Delivery: Focus on Quality

Arif Kamal, associate professor of medicine and population health sciences at the Duke University School of Medicine, began by reminding attendees that health care and society are both at an inflection point. Kamal said,

> There has been nothing more transformative than a global pandemic to remind us that quality of life is really important, regardless of whether we have a serious illness, take care of a loved one with a serious illness, or are at risk of a serious illness, and nothing more than a pandemic can remind us that we are all a very short way from having a serious illness if we do not have one right now.

What that means, he continued, is that the health care system and society need to be deliberate in their actions and steps to care for people with serious illness. This includes ensuring that people are honored as people first and patients second and that the health care system attends to caregivers' needs.

Palliative care, in Kamal's view, is starting to enter its third iteration. "Palliative care 1.0," as he called it, describes the first phase when health systems and society became aware that patients and caregivers suffer from both serious illness and the experience of dealing with the health care system. Other characteristics of the earlier phase included the realization by health systems that a focus on quality of life does not happen by accident but rather by design. This intentional focus involves paying attention to patient and caregiver needs, conducting meticulous assessments, putting teams around patients and their caregivers, and making sure that care teams remain in lockstep with patient and caregiver values and priorities to meet their goals of care.

"Palliative care 2.0," said Kamal, refers to when palliative care became more broadly available to populations with serious illness and attention was focused on ensuring that the services, standards, guidelines, quality measures, and clinical delivery mechanisms could meet their needs.

We are currently on the cusp of palliative care 3.0, explained Kamal, as palliative care transitions from availability to accessibility. "Availability is I have a service, accessibility is making sure the people that can benefit the most find these services and get regular interactions with them," he explained. Successfully making that transition, however, will require focusing on three critical areas: championing a workforce, developing quality measures in gap areas, and engaging and empowering patients and caregivers.

While palliative care is considered a medical specialty, the bottom line, said Kamal, is that the 7,000 or so specialists in the United States, along with countless nurses, social workers, chaplains, pharmacists, and other team members, cannot possibly meet the needs of all those with serious illness (Kamal et al., 2019). The future workforce situation is even more alarming; the number of palliative care physicians is expected to decrease over the next 20 years as that population ages at the same time that the demand for services is predicted to grow as a result of the entire U.S. population aging (Kamal et al., 2019). Kamal explained that there will be an untenable ratio of those who are eligible for palliative care services and those physicians who are available to serve that population. About 14 complex patients must be seen every single day per palliative care physician. This number is expected to rise to 22–23, which represents an impossible case load (Kamal et al., 2019).

To Kamal and his colleagues, the only solution is to embrace all members of the health care team as individuals dedicated to delivering palliative care services (Kamal et al., 2015, 2016). This approach features every single member delivering basic or fundamental palliative care. Moreover, it involves focusing on every person as an individual, recognizing that, as a person with serious illness, they face challenges related to their quality of life, and putting a plan in place to help them manage their illness and maintain quality of life.

Beyond the basic or fundamental palliative care is a second level of expertise that Kamal refers to as the "champions." This second level includes PCPs, hospitalists, intensivists, oncologists, and other team members who are interested in providing additional layers of support to patients, recognizing that areas of distress can come from many different sources and that complexity will be the norm. A third level includes palliative care specialists—the clinicians who have additional training through fellowships and other opportunities—caring for individuals who need the most specialized and perhaps most intensive interventions, said Kamal. He referred to the first workshop and Twaddle's reference to the fourth edition of the Clinical Practice Guidelines for Quality Palliative Care. As Twaddle explained, these guidelines are organized around eight domains of care that are relevant for any patient with serious illness and their caregivers, not only those receiving palliative care. Kamal acknowledged the widespread support these guidelines have received from the serious illness community and noted that the guidelines influenced the development of a measurement framework for palliative care by the National Quality Forum (NQF). It considers the types of palliative care, the settings in which it is delivered and the domains of care to be centered around the patient and family (see Figure 3).

Echoing themes raised in the first webinar, Kamal added that the NQF framework also includes finances as a domain of care, recogniz-

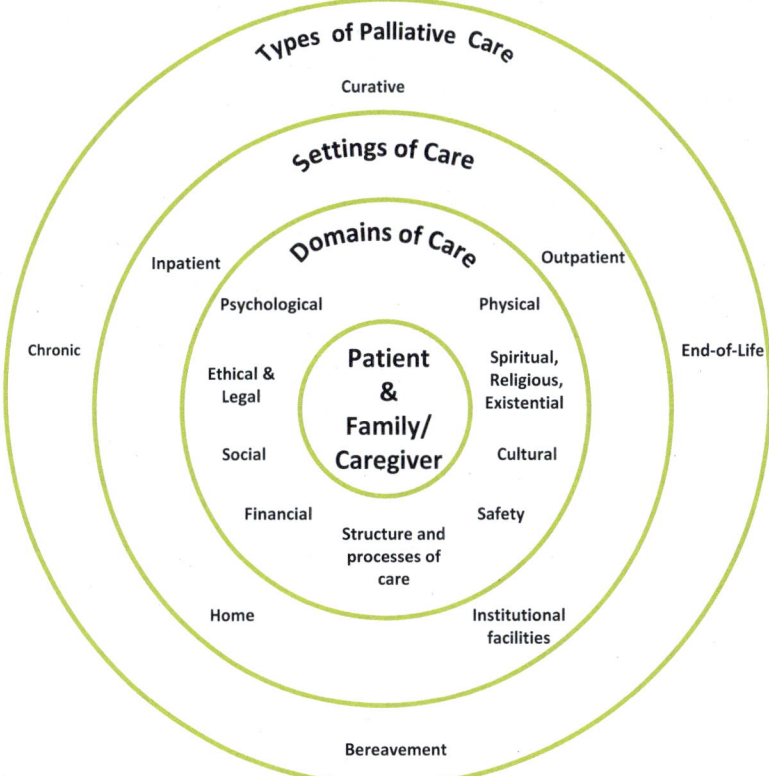

FIGURE 3 The National Quality Forum measurement framework for palliative care.
SOURCE: As presented by Arif Kamal, June 17, 2021.

ing that financial toxicity[24] is a significant component of low quality of life for patients with serious illness. Patients with advanced cancer, for example, will often drain their entire savings or declare bankruptcy. This untenable financial logistical complexity, he added, bleeds into every component of an individual's life and has a significant impact on their sense of personhood.

---

[24] "Financial toxicity describes problems a cancer patient has related to the cost of treatment. The terms financial toxicity and financial distress are used to describe how out-of-pocket costs can cause financial problems for a patient." For more information, see https://www.cancer.gov/about-cancer/managing-care/track-care-costs/financial-toxicity-pdq (accessed August 17, 2021).

Kamal and his colleagues looked at how the NQF measures mapped to the eight domains to identify opportunities for developing quality measures to help move the field forward into the 3.0 era (Kamal et al., 2014). They found many measures of the physical and structural aspects of care but fewer in the cultural, spiritual, and social aspects. He and his colleagues have since been thinking about expanded frameworks for quality measurement that would go beyond structure, process, and health outcomes to include access, resource use, experience, cost, and overall population health (Kamal et al., 2020).

Kamal highlighted the work of the Palliative Care Quality Collaborative,[25] which represents the first nationally unified effort to collect structure, process, and outcomes data that are patient specific but also relevant to the serious illness field and organizationally informative. The data come from the National Palliative Care Registry, the Palliative Care Quality Network, and the Global Palliative Care Quality Alliance, with funding from the Gordon and Betty Moore Foundation and the Cambia Health Foundation. The goal of this effort, he explained, is to improve the quality of palliative care delivery through a collaborative, learning-centered approach.

Kamal concluded by emphasizing the overarching importance of engaging people and family members in serious illness care. He also called attention to innovative approaches to fill current gaps in quality measurements.

The Centers for Medicare & Medicaid Services Innovation Center: Demonstration Projects to Support Comprehensive Care

The Centers for Medicare & Medicaid Services (CMS) Innovation Center, explained Amy Bassano, the center's deputy director, was created over a decade ago to test alternative, innovative payment and service delivery models to reduce cost, improve quality, and enhance patient-centered care. Since its inception, the Innovation Center has placed a high priority on models relevant to primary care and advanced care for patients with serious illness. She noted that its models have provided valuable insights to inform the design and development of subsequent models with common approaches. Early models supported enhanced and integrated care with minimal financial risk; newer models include higher standards in quality reporting, more opportunities for shared savings, and integration of clinical treatment and social services.

---

[25] For more information, see https://palliativequality.org (accessed August 17, 2021).

Bassano described the Comprehensive Primary Care Plus Model,[26] which was the center's second initiative that aimed to expand primary care services and integrate different types of services into primary care. It represents a move away from fee-for-service reimbursement and is beginning to produce small, favorable effects on the use of Medicare services, including reducing the rate of emergency department visits and increasing ambulatory primary care visits, said Bassano. She added that the model provided better incentives to care for patients with serious illness and refer them to the services they need.

The Primary Care First[27] model, launched at the beginning of 2021, includes payment options for practices able to accept increased financial risk in exchange for flexibility and potential rewards based on performance, including support for those serving high-needs populations. Bassano explained that participants can also select a "hybrid" option to simultaneously participate in both the primary care and high-needs population options. She added that the goals are to reduce Medicare spending by preventing avoidable hospital readmissions and to improve quality of and access to care for all Medicare beneficiaries, particularly those with complex chronic conditions and serious illness. Bassano noted that the second option has yet to be implemented, in large part because of the difficulty in identifying individuals who would benefit from this approach. "They have no one who is coordinating their care, but given some of the HIPAA protections and other beneficiary protections in the program, we cannot reach out to them and we cannot have third parties reach out to them," she explained.

Direct contracting in one of the center's newest models offers new forms of capitated, population-based payments, enhanced payment options, and flexibilities to increase the tools available to meet Medicare beneficiaries' medical and nonmedical needs. Bassano explained that the goals are to transform risk-sharing arrangements in fee-for-service Medicare, empower beneficiaries to personally engage in their own care delivery, and reduce provider burden to meet health care needs effectively. This model also has a high-needs track that includes appropriate risk adjustment and other payment methodologies. Bassano noted that six organizations spanning 12 states are participating in the high-needs track.

---

[26] For more information, see https://innovation.cms.gov/innovation-models/comprehensive-primary-care-plus (accessed August 17, 2021).

[27] For more information, see https://innovation.cms.gov/innovation-models/primary-care-first-model-options (accessed August 17, 2021).

Bassano also described one of the center's older models, the Medicare Care Choices Model.[28] It allows Medicare beneficiaries who qualify for hospice to receive supportive care services while receiving care for their terminal condition. Bassano explained that evidence from the private market shows that concurrent care can improve outcomes, ameliorate patient and family experiences, and lower costs. Hospices are paid $200 or $400 if the beneficiary is enrolled for less than 15 days or 15 or more days in a calendar month, respectively. More than 80 hospices are participating in this program, which will end in 2021.[23] Bassano remarked that the most recent evaluation found that the program was successful in lowering costs, but the results were not generalizable because of the limited number of participants.

CMS is continuing to test how Medicare Advantage (MA)[29] organizations can better target supplemental benefit design based on chronic conditions and/or socioeconomic characteristics through the MA Value Based Insurance Design (VBID) model. Prior to the launch of VBID, MA patients had to disenroll from the MA program if they needed hospice services. The program has 14 participants in 30 states and Puerto Rico, with the goal to expand VBID in 2022.[24] Bassano pointed out the effective collaboration between hospices and MA plans on how to model the work given the vulnerability of these patients.

Going forward, Bassano and her colleagues are looking at how to continue to develop models that serve those with serious illness in a manner that is patient-centered and addresses disparities in health. In closing, Bassano emphasized that the goal is to apply the lessons from tested models to continue efforts to improve care and access to care.

Congressional Action to Improve Care for People with Serious Illness

Megan Thompson, senior policy advisor in the office of Senator Jacky Rosen (D-NV), provided an update on legislative action related to serious illness care. Thompson explained that Senator Rosen is founder and co-chair of the Senate's bipartisan Comprehensive Care Caucus, which focuses on palliative care, care coordination, and support for caregivers. The inspira-

---

[28] For more information, see https://innovation.cms.gov/innovation-models/medicare-care-choices (accessed August 17, 2021).

[29] For more information, see https://www.medicare.gov/sign-up-change-plans/types-of-medicare-health-plans/medicare-advantage-plans (accessed August 17, 2021).

tion for the caucus evolved from Senator Rosen's experience caring for her parents and in-laws at the ends of their lives and her frustrations accessing comprehensive care services, Thompson added.

Thompson explained that in many areas of Nevada, access to certain types of specialty care necessitate driving long distances. To consider ways to expand access to care, Thompson and her colleagues began talking with physicians and community health centers throughout the state. They learned that there was a great need for ongoing medical training opportunities for clinicians to enable them to better serve the most vulnerable patients without requiring them to physically bring in a specialist who might not even exist in their part of the state.

Based on what was learned from these discussions, Senator Rosen introduced the Improving Access to Health Care in Rural and Underserved Areas Act[30] with Senator Lisa Murkowski (R-AK), which has two components. The first part would fund specialists through grants with community health centers and rural health clinics based on the needs that they identify given their patient population, explained Thompson. Under the terms of the bill, access could be virtual or in person depending on logistics. Appointments would be held jointly with the patient's PCP. She added that the idea is to ensure a comprehensive patient experience and that the PCP has a learning opportunity that counts toward their continuing education requirement.

Thompson noted that Senator Rosen led a successful bipartisan effort to recognize November as National Hospice and Palliative Care Month. The accompanying resolution, which passed by unanimous consent, referred to palliative care as complementary to curative treatments and emphasized the benefits of integrating it early into the treatment plans for patients with serious illness or injury.

Thompson and her colleagues are working on two additional bills that focus on improving palliative care for seniors enrolled in Medicare. The provisions in the first of these bills would build on efforts at CMS to support community-based palliative care and allow access to care as close as possible to the time of diagnosis. This would ideally improve outcomes and quality of life. Thompson explained that the second bill aims to address barriers for patients with serious illness who require regular transfusions, such as those with leukemia, lymphoma, and sickle cell disease. In closing, Thompson noted that this bill would create a mechanism to pay for trans-

---

[30] For more information, see https://www.congress.gov/bill/116th-congress/senate-bill/3194/text (accessed August 17, 2021).

fusions without requiring the patient to be in hospice care but still allow hospice benefits when needed.

Palliative Care and Serious Disease Management in Primary Care

In the session's final presentation, Adam Barde, senior director for Health Transformation Implementation at Blue Shield of California, and Kimberly Bower, medical director for the Blue Shield of California Promise Health Plan, discussed how Blue Shield of California is incorporating palliative care and serious disease management into primary care. This effort, explained Barde, recognizes the many challenges that the nation's health care system faces, including unsustainable cost, patient and provider dissatisfaction, poor health outcomes and health inequities. Addressing this long list of problems, he added, requires investing in primary care. Barde remarked that such an investment should provide increased time for physicians to engage in shared decision making with their patients, incorporate community-integrated health services, and integrate an improved model of palliative care into care delivery.

Referencing the triple aim and quadruple aim[31] frameworks that are helping to drive health care system reform, Barde explained that his organization's philosophy is built on the quintuple aim recognizing the importance of increasing health equity and the provider experience. The result, said Barde, is the organization's Health Reimagined[32] practice transformation solutions that include:

1. Shared decision making that improves patient engagement and satisfaction by empowering patients to actively participate in their care planning and treatment;
2. Virtual care that establishes a platform for real-time virtual interaction between patients and their regular health professionals for diagnosis, treatment, and management of medical conditions;

---

[31] The triple aim includes improving the patient experience of care, improving the health of populations, and reducing per capita costs of health care. The quadruple aim also includes improving the clinician experience. For more information, see https://www.ncbi.nlm.nih.gov/pmc/articles/PMC4226781 (accessed August 17, 2021).

[32] For more information, see https://healthreimagined.blueshieldca.com (accessed September 20, 2021).

3. Community health advocates who work with, or on behalf of, patients to navigate the health system and connect them with community resources that address their social needs and reduce health inequities; and
4. Real-time claims settlement using direct connection digital solutions that enhances the speed of claims processes from days to seconds.

Barde explained that as both a payer and part of the health care delivery system, Blue Shield of California believes it is imperative to support primary care in new ways through innovative payment models. Barde pointed out that one such model includes value-based payments combined with per member per month payments to support key activities that occur both during and outside of the traditional office visit, including care coordination, testing, and referrals to palliative care and hospice programs. Barde explained that the model rewards proactive outreach to other home- and community-based clinical services that can include coordinating of care with a home-based palliative care team. Blue Shield of California is also adjusting payments based on service intensity and providing additional revenue opportunities tied to quality as defined by HEDIS measures, resource use measures, and member satisfaction scores.

Bower discussed Blue Shield of California's view of palliative care as a continuum—one that starts early in a patient's experience with serious illness. This view, combined with the Health Reimagined initiative, is designed to help PCPs have the time and space to delivery primary level palliative care in their office, which would include symptom management and time to discuss both primary care and ACP. Currently, a PCP can bill for a palliative care consultation, but that would not constitute true team-based palliative care. She added that not funding an interdisciplinary care team means that patients have difficulty accessing essential palliative care services. In an ideal world, said Bower, when a primary care provider needs help from a specialist, they would refer their patient to clinic-based palliative care.

Bower's organization has also created a payment model for pre-hospice, home-based palliative care designed to provide subspecialty level palliative care and be an extension of the primary care office into the home for those who are at risk of dying in the next year and have the following:

- Significant functional impairment that limits their ability to get to in-person care;

- Social determinants that cannot be addressed effectively in the office and that interfere with optimal care; or
- Struggles with adherence to the treatment plan.

Bower added that each care team must have a medical director and a spiritual counselor, be able to do consultations at home, and provide 24/7 telephone support. Members do not pay copays or co-insurance for services, and home-based palliative care providers are paid a monthly case rate.

Early results for this initiative include establishing of a statewide network of palliative care providers, though in some remote areas, services are only available virtually. Since its inception in 2017, 3,064 members have enrolled, with 52 percent completing advance directives and 90 percent designating a durable power of attorney for health care. Bower shared that internal program data show approximately 20 percent of the enrollees enter into hospice care, 10 percent die while in the program, and about 70 percent stabilize, and for some, transition out of the program. Others may leave the program due to changes in insurance.

Bower explained that the unpublished claims data indicate that per member, per month costs for emergency department use and hospitalizations have fallen, with the median expenditure dropping from $1,204 per member per month to $45, and the mean dropping from $3,996 per member per month to $2,746. She added that inpatient visits have fallen from 1,255 per thousand members to 1,069 and emergency department visits went from 1,034 per 1,000 members to 851. Bower noted that most of the cost savings support the payments for the program's providers and its administrative costs and internal surveys show that the majority of members are satisfied or very satisfied with the program; most common negative comments are about things that are not included in the palliative care package, such as a home health aide. She added that one area that needs improvement is the communication between the PCP and the freestanding community-based palliative care provider.

To conclude, Bower focused on future directions for home-based palliative care in primary care. She explained that she and her colleagues believe there is a gap in the provision of clinic-based palliative care. Blue Shield of California is working on payment models that will provide a case rate along with a value-based incentive to support an interdisciplinary palliative care team in the clinic setting. "We also think that we need to support our primary care doctors in shared decision making by giving them extra time with patients, and access to cloud-based tools that help patients prepare before conversations with their provider," said Bower. These shared decision-making modules, she noted, should be a resource for PCPs that can help them integrate elements of palliative care earlier in serious disease management. In closing, Bower observed that as health care systems move away from paying for volume to paying for value, integration of palliative care into the care delivery model will be essential.

Discussion

Rodgers opened the discussion session by asking Olex to comment on the things about the health care system, teams, and interactions that he would change to make his experience more patient-centered and responsive to his needs. Olex replied that he would like primary care to be able to advise him on steps he can take to make a difference in his own life in terms of exercises, stretching activities, and dietary changes so that he would not have to see a specialist for every aspect of his care. In addition, he would like to have more open conversations with his PCPs that lead to more comprehensive care that goes beyond dealing specifically with his multiple sclerosis.

Rodgers then asked Thompson to elaborate on what she and Senator Rosen hope the legislation discussed earlier could accomplish. Thompson replied that one goal is to provide increased support and education for PCPs to enable them to provide better care for their patients without having to refer patients to specialists. Over the long term, this would both enhance primary care and provide more direct access to the services that specialty and palliative care can deliver, while also helping physicians meet their continuing medical education requirements. Rodgers commented that this approach could be part of a portfolio of solutions that respond to the needs of different clinical scenarios and different communities.

Rodgers then invited the speakers to comment on the challenges they have encountered while trying to implement the value-based payment models necessary for supporting primary care and palliative care integration. Bassano replied that CMS's statutory framework requires a model to save money and/or improve quality. For voluntary participation models, CMS looks at selection effects and how the model can attract a variety of different participants and evaluate the model as it pertains to its statutory requirements. She noted that the Innovation Center runs more than 40 models and needs to differentiate where one model ends and another begins as a way of reducing the number of interventions. Rodgers commented on the difficulty of trying to prove a model will save money before testing it and that he appreciates the work CMS has put into that.

Barde said that his organization wanted to develop a payment model that would allow physicians and providers to practice medicine in the way they had been trained, which requires moving to a value-based model that enables physicians to engage in the needed conversations with their patients. The two key challenges his organization has faced have physician adoption of the model, which Barde attributes to their lack of trust in payers, and adopting a payment model for a limited portion of Blue Shield of California's line of business due to regulatory constraints. In Barde's view, the best approach would be to have all payers become part of these models so that practices could modify their procedures and workloads for all of their patients.

Bower remarked that a fundamental constraint to developing a new model is the need to ensure that it does not lead to increased premiums. Bower pointed out that a significant impediment to implementation is the lack of billing codes to pay for interdisciplinary palliative care. Another challenge is the need for quality data given that these models pay for quality. Bower explained that despite the great deal of quality data available, most of the data are not accessible through the claims system. Instead, they rely on physician-reported quality data, which again raises the trust issue. Barde added that the lack of interoperability among EHR systems is another impediment to model adoption.

Rodgers thanked the speakers for talking about quality of care because that often is lost when the focus is largely on reducing costs. He also pointed to the interoperability challenge as one that confounds physicians and patients alike. Rodgers then asked Kamal for his ideas on how to ensure high-quality serious illness care regardless of how providers are paid. Kamal endorsed the idea of the quintuple aim and its need for a broad scale patient-reported outcome performance measure that is generated immediately. This will enable the creation of a learning health system that is agile and able to improve continuously based on real-time, patient-reported data on quality of care. Kamal also would like to see a measure that encompasses both caregiver and financial toxicity and caregiver needs. Kamal called for serious consideration for the issue of out-of-pocket costs that represent a significant barrier to care for many patients. Rodgers noted that Blue Shield of California's model tackles this last issue by eliminating copays and co-insurance for participants of its home-based palliative care model.

Bassano remarked that the CMS Innovation Center sees a great deal of promise in a palliative care model that has the flexibility to test adding benefits in a way that should improve quality and be cost neutral, as in the CMS model that added diabetes prevention. Bassano added that CMS has been sensitive to adding benefits that will increase costs for beneficiaries, and Kamal noted that the paucity of data on the financial toxicity of palliative care and the need for regular visits. He pointed out that some trials of new models have difficulty recruiting participants because people do not want to be in the group with regular commercial insurance copay. "It is important to recognize that even the delivery of these great services that we are talking about can introduce financial toxicity, and exploring all the different ways to ameliorate that is important," said Kamal.

Several audience members asked about lessons from Blue Shield of California's experience that could influence how its model is implemented elsewhere and, in particular, if it felt that engaging a vendor to help them recruit participants was useful. Bower replied that the program no longer contracts with an outreach vendor because it was not productive. Without engaging primary care, she added, it is difficult to identify those who would benefit from palliative care given the limitations of claims data to reveal functional status or social determinants. "I feel pretty strongly at this point that we need to partner with our PCPs and our subspecialists and our hospitalists to identify those patients and get them referred," Bower said. Barde added that the program is trying to use data from multiple sources, both internal and external, to power outreach efforts. Blue Shield of California is testing an approach that engages community health advocates in efforts to identify patient needs before they become more severe.

To conclude the session, Rodgers asked the speakers to identify the main priorities to ensure access to high-quality serious illness care. Bower and Barde said a key priority is to expand the acceptance of palliative care beyond the majority white population by building trust among minority and vulnerable populations. They noted that Blue Shield of California is working to engage community health advocates in that trust-building activity.

Bassano noted that CMS also views increasing access to and use of palliative care services among minority and underserved populations as top priorities. Accomplishing that goal will require models that address diverse populations, involve diverse type of providers, and work in partnership with communities and the people the models are intended to serve. Kamal commented that he and his collaborators are trying to be precise about how they collect demographic data on those they serve as a means of identifying the serious illness and palliative care needs of particular populations and matching them with the appropriate services.

Thompson pointed to the importance of bringing health care to where the people are, perhaps via mobile clinics. She noted that Senator Rosen is working on legislation that would provide some flexibility within funding streams so that community health centers could be as creative as possible in terms of reaching out and bringing care to people with issues in access, which would also address equity. She also pointed out the need to increase the number of people working in health care and the importance of encouraging students from all communities to pursue careers in the health sciences.

In the final comments of the session, Olex remarked that peer coordination has been important in the multiple sclerosis community. He wondered, given privacy and regulatory concerns, if it would be possible to bring more patients into the system as peer advisors.

PROMISING INTEGRATED CARE MODELS

Serious Illness Conversations in Federally Qualified Health Centers

The workshop's final session began with a presentation from Deborah Swiderski, associate professor of medicine and family and social medicine at the Albert Einstein College of Medicine and a primary care internist at the Montefiore Medical Center, on efforts to integrate serious illness care into two FQHCs. In 2018, Swiderski and her collaborators received funding from Ariadne Labs[33] to support implementing serious illness conversation training in two FQHCs in the Bronx, New York, using Ariadne's Serious Illness Conversation Guide,[34] a checklist approach to embedding this work in clinical practice. Swiderski noted that much of the work to explore its effectiveness had been conducted in well-resourced sites serving primarily white, well-insured patients. In contrast, Swiderski explained, FQHCs often serve patients in communities affected by poverty, a lack of adequate insurance, and health disparities that lead to the complex presentation of chronic illnesses. FQHCs typically are overburdened, underresourced, and highly stressed clinical settings observed Swiderski.

Swiderski and her colleagues trained 15 family medicine attending physicians and 4 nurses at the two FQHCs. Of the 15 physicians, 11 had 37 conversations using the guide over a 6-month period according to inter-

---

[33] For more information, see https://www.ariadnelabs.org (accessed August 17, 2021).

[34] The guide is available free-of-charge at https://www.ariadnelabs.org/wp-content/uploads/2017/05/SI-CG-2017-04-21_FINAL.pdf (accessed August 17, 2021).

nal data. Swiderski's team then interviewed these 11 physicians about their experience using the guide and compiled a list of lessons learned. One lesson was the importance of assembling the right team for implementation, which in this case included several PCPs working in FQHCs who could provide deep, experiential knowledge about the environment that they were trying to influence. Swiderski shared that she has 20 years of experience teaching this material to residents. In fact, she said, a great strength of the implementation team was that the members brought complementary skill sets to the effort and everyone involved shared a strong sense of mission.

As the project's clinical lead, Swiderski made a point of engaging personally with all stakeholders as a way to promote buy-in to the program. "I met with executive directors, medical directors, nursing leadership, and site personnel, social workers, and primary care providers," explained Swiderski. "I made short presentations at team meetings, I wrangled a family medicine grand rounds, and I used these not just to present what the project was, but as opportunities for informal needs assessment, which is crucial." Most importantly, Swiderski and her team made sure to schedule training sessions at already scheduled meeting times, so that there was no additional time commitment required from the FQHCs already overburdened with primary care providers.

Swiderski noted that coaching and support after formal training are essential. She explained that funding was limited in the initial phase, so the project suffered from a lack of coaching and support, but a project manager now helps to organize and implement this aspect. Swiderski emphasized that coaching should be at the individual provider level and in groups, such as during grand rounds and via programmatic-level reminders and refreshers, such as newsletters.

Swiderski explained that creating a one-size-fits-all solution does not work. Rather, the approach "has to emerge from the site itself." Swiderski added that she could not overstate the importance of a site champion, which her program was fortunate to identify. They help maintain momentum and can play a significant role in coaching and supporting staff and also serve a critical role in figuring out site-specific workflows. Currently, the champions are not compensated with either funding or time, so she and her colleagues have made it a point to ensure their dedication to the work is rewarded with extra training and support to help them build their knowledge base made the work much easier. "We found that trying to get primary care providers to use a checklist was a matter of culture change, but ultimately [they felt it was] helpful. The numerous barriers in doing this work in these settings were truly tempered by the affirmation of the importance of relationship-based care," she said. "This work has meaning, but these barriers are real and will require systems change for large-scale implementation to occur." She concluded her remarks with a quote from one of the project's site champions: "having a serious illness conversation with your patient is not extra work, it's learning to do what we already do better. Serious illness conversations help to improve the way we see our patients."

The ChenMed Model of Care

Faisel Syed, national director for primary care at ChenMed, opened by recounting how his father was seen by multiple specialists to treat his heart disease, diabetes, lower back pain, and memory loss. Syed pointed out that his father's care was uncoordinated and ineffective; he was taking medications to counter the side effects from other medications because his specialists failed to communicate with one another. Syed explained that eventually he was able to convince his father to enroll in an MA program with a PCP who would coordinate his care. Though his father was initially skeptical, today, his heart function is normal, his diabetes is controlled, and his back pain and memory loss are gone. "When we talk about delivering high-quality, integrated primary care for serious illness, I think about Dad and others like him," explained Syed.

In Syed's view, one problem with the U.S. health care system is that it pays doctors on a fee-for-service basis that leads to them spending too much time worrying about relative value units and suffering from what Syed referred to as "transaction distraction." ChenMed operates on a full-cost, value-based care model which, in contrast, focuses on improving the quality of care, patient and provider satisfaction, and saving money, noted Syed. He observed that achieving this quadruple aim starts with acknowledging that the doctor–patient relationship is sacred, the doctor-to-doctor relationship is congenial and collaborative, and the doctor–staff relationship is courteous and codependent. "You cannot have integrated care without integrated relationships," said Syed.

Syed explained that ChenMed physicians give their mobile phone numbers to their patients. If Syed needs help getting his patient to adhere to a treatment plan, he will call their children and grandchildren for backup. Patients, Syed explained, receive a daily text about health such as reminders to get a flu shot or to stay hydrated on a hot summer day. ChenMed care teams call their patients weekly, even if they are healthy, and see them in person at least monthly to prevent small problems from growing. "Anyone can learn the pathophysiology it takes to keep people healthy, but the knowledge is useless if your patients do not trust you," noted Syed. "When there is trust between the doctor and the patient, it can then create achievable goals that lead to better health." Trust, he added, can lead to something else—discussions about end-of-life wishes that come naturally.

Syed pointed out that the model he described works with any patient; he explained that ChenMed patients are some of the most underserved people in the United States. He described the ChenMed model of care as a throwback to a different era of medicine—one that considers the entire patient and gets to know them and what the nonmedical aspects of their lives could be affecting their health. Syed pointed out that this model has been implemented successfully in cities of all sizes and continued spreading during the pandemic. "We keep growing because the model keeps us profitable. In the high-touch, integrated, value-based care model, the savings are 30 percent with 50 percent fewer hospitalizations" said Syed (Ghany et al., 2018).

The United States, said Syed, claims to have the world's best health care system and many patients with complex disease do receive remarkable care. However, if access is limited by income, then improving health care for all becomes difficult. This country also claims to have the world's best medical education system, but those clinicians who go into primary care are financially punished for it when they also have to deal with a quarter of a million dollars in medical school debt, he added. "Primary care doctors are supposed to be at the center of the health care delivery model and are supposed to be the gateway to better health, not the gatekeeper to medication refills and referrals. Debt has diminished the role of primary care," in Syed's view. "We are suffering from a shortage of primary care doctors, and that will not change until we level the compensation playing field," he added.

For Syed, solving the nation's health care problems requires looking at the bigger picture, and the way to transition to a high-quality integrated primary care model is to pay for quality instead of transactions. "Any time you mess with people's money, you are going to get pushback, but we must start paying for better health, rather than transactions," said Syed in closing. "Doctors and insurance companies must work together, and switch the goal from billing to well-being and rewarding doctors for making people healthier. Transactions do not lead to better health; they only lead to more transactions," he concluded.

Transforming Urgent Care for Veterans with Serious Illness

Thomas Edes, senior medical advisor for geriatrics and extended care at the U.S. Department of Veterans Affairs (VA), discussed the VA's transformation of urgent and emergent care for veterans with serious, chronic, and disabling conditions. He opened his remarks by identifying three key elements of successful change in health care:

1. The power of persistence,
2. The importance of serendipity, and
3. The importance of collaboration in creating meaningful change.

Edes noted that the VA's transformation of urgent and emergent care for older veterans was sparked by a convergence of problems and solutions. The problems, he said, were likely familiar to all workshop participants. They included a worsening of the health care workforce shortage and an increasing population of older Americans with serious chronic diseases and unmet needs tied to the social determinants of health, fragmented care, and an unsustainable rise in health care costs (Edes, 2019; Foley and Luz, 2021). At the VA, the solutions included the rise of interdisciplinary teams, person-centered care, age-friendly health systems, intermediate care technicians who arrived with incredible skills after serving as military medics and corpsmen, and coordination and collaboration among emergency medicine, geriatrics, and primary care.

Edes recounted the case of an 87-year-old man with heart disease, hypertension, and other medical issues who was discharged to home after hospitalization for a change in cognition arising from a possible stroke. Multiple family members worked hard to help him, but none were able to remain with him at all times. About 17 days later he was back in the emergency department after a fall. The emergency department crew quickly addressed his urgent medical needs and determined he was medically stable.

Edes explained that given that it was a geriatric emergency department, an additional screening that identified this person as a senior at risk. As a result, he was seen by an interdisciplinary team that included the emergency department social worker, a physical therapist, and a pharmacist. The team identified significant unmet needs that would likely complicate his ability to remain at home, so they altered the care plan to address balance and gait difficulties, perform a home safety evaluation, eliminate potentially inappropriate medications, and provide some caregiver support, durable medical equipment for home use, and home supportive services. The result, said Edes, was a successful discharge to home after a short stay in rehabilitative care.

Edes explained that the VA transformation effort was triggered by a few timely and unpredictable events. After Hurricane Katrina, one of the VA's national senior executive leaders chose to step down from his position and go to New Orleans to help rebuild the health care systems. One day, Edes recalled, this individual called him and said he wanted New Orleans to become the exemplary care model for older veterans, and asked if Edes would help. Edes was eager to do so; he took a quick trip to New Orleans to talk to the leaders of a variety of geriatric and palliative care programs and other department leaders, including the director of the New Orleans VA emergency department. The director explained to Edes that too many older veterans with serious chronic diseases who show up in her department end up hospitalized merely because it is not safe for them to go home.

Upon his return to Washington, DC, Edes called the VA's national director of emergency medicine and the transformation project began, with the VA's office of geriatrics and extended care making it a strategic priority to implement age-friendly health systems standard throughout the VA. The transformation initiative launched on February 4, 2020, with the first cohort of 20 VA emergency departments that volunteered. "They wanted to change their practices and wanted to go for geriatric emergency department accreditation," said Edes.

Edes explained that they then developed critical collaborations with a number of organizations, including The John A. Hartford Foundation, the West Health Institute, the American College of Emergency Physicians, the Geriatric Emergency Department Collaborative, and the VA Geriatric Research, Education, and Clinical Centers. Despite the COVID-19 pandemic striking 1 month later, that first cohort pressed on with their transformation, driven by their desire to better treat the high prevalence of older veterans with multiple chronic conditions who arrive in the emergency department and to increase the proportion who are discharged safely to home.

Edes explained that by May 2021, despite the worst pandemic in a century, 12 of the sites had achieved accreditation as geriatric emergency departments from the American College of Emergency Physicians[35] and the other 8 had their applications in review. Edes's office was overwhelmed

---

[35] For more information, see https://www.acep.org (accessed August 17, 2021).

by the number of additional sites that wanted to join. Currently, 32 additional VA emergency departments and 1 urgent care center are undergoing their own transformations, which would mean that nearly half the 110 VA emergency departments will be part of this initiative. In addition, several in the first cohort are now aiming to become Level 2 or Level 1 geriatric emergency departments, explained Edes (Castellucci, 2018).

Edes noted that the VA program aligns patient goals of care with their care plan and increases continuity with primary care. As a result, the total cost of care has fallen as care has shifted from the emergency department and the hospital to home, with a corresponding increase in addressing previously unmet needs for personal care and palliative care (Cornell et al., 2020; Huded et al., 2020; Hwang and Morrison, 2007; Hwang et al., 2021; Tinetti et al., 2021).

Edes recounted another case in which an 85-year-old presented to the emergency department after a fall. Upon determining that he was medically stable, he was referred to the department's social worker, who felt that the veteran was not fully disclosing some of his concerns. The intermediate care technician, a former military medic, stepped in. Because of the immediate bond of trust between the two veterans, the man confessed that he was struggling to take care of himself at home, he was depressed, and his wife of 60 years had recently been placed in a nursing facility. What he really wanted was to be reunited with his wife. Staff arranged for him to be moved into her nursing home. While this did not fit with the initiative's goal to shift care to the home and reduce costs, it did meet his needs, and that is what matters most, emphasized Edes.

Edes then listed a number of actions every emergency department could take immediately:

1. Evaluate your emergency department and determine what percentage of the individuals it is serving are over age 65, are hospitalized, and return to the emergency department within 30 days;
2. Identify seniors at risk and refer them to a primary care social worker;
3. Identify potentially inappropriate medications and refer patients to primary care;
4. Convene champions in primary care, geriatrics, emergency medicine, palliative care, social work, and pharmacy;
5. Start small by connecting a primary care social worker or nurse coordinator with a local emergency department; start with one shift per week, or daily check in at 4 pm;

6. Pursue Level 3 American College of Emergency Physicians Geriatric Emergency Department Accreditation;
7. Explore age-friendly healthy systems and "geriatrics plus" care, initiating a collaboration between a geriatric clinic or home care with primary care or between geriatrics and emergency medicine; and
8. Work with the Institute for Healthcare Improvement[36] to integrate "what matters" into practice by training, tracking, and providing feedback on discussing and incorporating "what matters" or patient goals into health record and care plan.

As far as what is next for the VA, Edes said he and his colleagues are working on developing a mobile workforce that is coordinated with the emergency department and community collaborative partners. The goal, he said, is to avoid trips to the emergency department whenever possible. "We are excited with where we are in VA and where we are going in VA, and we are eager to continue learning from and working with others on this journey," said Edes in closing.

The CARIÑOS Approach: Caring for Persons with Serious Illness

In the workshop's final presentation, Neela K. Patel, Joe R. and Teresa Lozano Long Chair in Community Geriatrics and Senior Care and associate professor and chief of geriatrics and supportive care at University of Texas Health San Antonio, discussed the CARIÑOS approach to care that her institution started developing in 2010. Patel explained that, in Spanish, CARIÑOS means tenderness, fondness, and love. Patel noted that the division of geriatrics and supportive care serves approximately 3,500 individuals—64 percent Hispanic and 25 percent living in underserved communities—in various clinical settings, including nursing homes, assisted living facilities, and independent living, and it has a hospital-based consult service in geriatrics and palliative care according to internal organization data. As a result of the COVID-19 pandemic and the isolation that patients were experiencing, the practice has become 50 percent ambulatory visits and 50 percent home visits.

The CARIÑOS approach is based on seven key principles:

---

[36] For more information, see http://www.ihi.org (accessed August 17, 2021).

1. **C**omprehensive, coordinated, compassionate care across various clinical settings that meets older adults' needs beyond the office walls.
2. **A**dvocating for patients and families by collaborating and maintaining relationships with other clinicians and health care partners.
3. **R**especting what matters most to older patients, such as meals, mobility, money, and medicines.
4. **I**ntentional activities and processes in the practice that are specific to meet the needs of older adults.
5. **N**urtured relationships with families, social service agencies, and community partners.
6. **O**lder adults are wise and know what they want, so listen to what they say.
7. **S**upportive care that focuses on quality of life.

The program started in the ambulatory setting, and it soon integrated what occurs in the clinic with the institution's hospital service. In fact, the clinic can admit patients to the hospital without going through the emergency department, Patel explained. She added that communication between the hospitalists and clinic staff has been good and enabled productive follow-ups regarding medication changes and care plans. The program has also collaborated with skilled and acute rehabilitation centers, further enhancing continuity of care. "We were talking to one another, we gave our cell phone number to one another for easier access, and we had access to the medical records from various places so that we could review the records for the patient," said Patel.

CARIÑOS also collaborated with home health and hospice agencies, improving communication and continuity of care which has led to in-service training opportunities for her primary care staff. "We put a lot on the primary care physician to coordinate," said Patel, "but this approach to care identifies roles and responsibilities for every person who is caring for the patient and family." She added that while the health care system is good at focusing on physical health, these older patients need care for their mental, emotional, and spiritual health. In her view, these health outcomes are ultimately more crucial than their physical health outcomes.

Patel's team has identified resources that the program can draw upon to meet these other needs. For example, the clinic did not have an on-staff social worker when it started, so the program collaborated with a social work agency that worked virtually and pro bono. Today, the clinic does have an embedded social worker on staff. Her team has also worked with durable medical equipment companies and transport agencies to improve patient access to supplies and the means to get to the clinic. Specialists and consultants are available when needed, but patients are encouraged not to make any changes to their care plan without working with a PCP; this ensures that everyone is on the same page.

Patel explained that focus group interviews revealed that the term "palliative care" was problematic in the Hispanic community because it was understood as giving up and not caring. Instead, she uses "supportive care" to be more culturally respectful and appropriate. This sensitivity to language has led to greater acceptance of supportive care consultations. Nonetheless, concluded Patel, the program was not reaching enough people, so she and her colleagues are now building culturally appropriate bridges to the community by working with professionally trained *promotores* (community health workers) to better understand the barriers that matter most to this community.

Discussion

Session moderator Lars Peterson, vice president of research at the American Board of Family Medicine, opened by asking the speakers to describe how they have made each of their programs financially sustainable. Syed replied that the main driver of waste in the U.S. health care system is unnecessary hospitalizations, which are fueled by unnecessary emergency department visits. Restoring the doctor–patient and doctor–doctor relationships and getting rid of the billing department[37] by assuming all patient costs has allowed ChenMed's providers to move care upstream, which keeps people out of the emergency department and the hospital. Swiderski said her program has been established for long enough to demonstrate that it is financially sustainable. Patel said her program's plan is to use the money it saves to integrate *promotores* into the model of care given the important cultural role they can play with the communities her institution services. She informs administrators that while the program may spend more on home health, it is keeping patients out of the emergency department and

---

[37] For more information, see https://topdoctormagazine.com/research/news/revolutionizing-the-american-healthcare-system-with-dr-faisel-syed-from-chenmed (accessed November 10, 2021).

saving money for the institution as a whole. She noted, too, that during the worst parts of the COVID-19 pandemic, her program was sustaining itself and actually doing better financially than it was before.

Edes noted that it is important when speaking with financial officers to remember that the typical profit margin is about 4 percent (Buttorff et al., 2017), which means that when a $10,000 hospitalization is avoided, the hospital only loses $400 rather than the entire $10,000. Moreover, patients and families speak to one another, and providing high-quality, coordinated primary care leads to more word-of-mouth referrals that can boost business and revenues. Finally, Edes noted that 50 percent of the nation's health care expenditures go to about 10 percent of the population, most of whom have a chronic, serious, disabling condition. Therefore, high-quality care for those individuals can make a significant dent in the U.S. health care spending (Buttorff et al., 2017).

Peterson asked the speakers for their thoughts on how their geriatric programs could be applied to pediatric palliative care. Patel replied that geriatrics and pediatrics involve similar strategies and that University of Texas Health has used the CARIÑOS model for its pediatric population. Swiderski said that the checklist approach her program uses to have end-of-life discussions with older adults could work well with pediatricians, for whom such conversations are incredibly difficult.

Syed was asked to elaborate on ChenMed's patient and clinician satisfaction outcomes and whether its approach could be expanded to noncapitated settings. Syed responded that he did not think it would be possible given the many restrictions tied to a noncapitated payment model. He noted that ChenMed had to develop its own EHR because the existing EHRs were designed for billing and referral purposes. "We needed a simple, effective EHR that was doctor-friendly," he said. Syed pointed out that ChenMed is in the top 10 percent on HEDIS and patient satisfaction scores. Sayed also shared that ChenMed did an internal company analysis and found physicians who have vaccinated 97 percent of their patients against influenza, even in the most vaccine-hesitant regions of the country. He credited the success rate to the trusting relationships that develop between ChenMed's patients and doctors.

Shifting the focus to the challenges of working in an emergency department, Peterson asked Edes how the VA's geriatric emergency department balances the need to get patients in and out as quickly as possible with the time that it takes to conduct the geriatric assessments that are an important part of the program. Edes replied that while they are still learning from their experiences, the data look good as far as maintaining that balance. This is in large part because the interdisciplinary team can quickly identify issues that help get people out of the waiting room and the emergency department faster.

For a final question, Peterson asked Swiderski how patients have reacted to the checklist. She replied that she recently received foundation funding to study that topic. At the time of the workshop, she said that her organization's physicians had reported that visits involving the checklist were meaningful for both them and their patients, and the patients frequently thanked them for those discussions. She noted that patients often want to have these conversations and that physicians believe they are important, but it is still necessary to document that the checklist provides a good experience for patients. As a final comment, Swiderski said that having these conversations are not about dying, but rather about living well with the time a person has left.

CLOSING REMARKS

After thanking all speakers and moderators, Rodgers provided a brief reflection about the workshop. The goal, he said, was to elevate the conversation about how to improve the experience that patients with serious illness encounter throughout their medical journey. To that end, the workshop began by highlighting the close and interlocking principles that underlie both specialty palliative care and primary care as laid out in the National Consensus Project Guidelines and the shared principles of primary care.

Next, the workshop highlighted the foundational importance of the interdisciplinary team in delivering that care. "What we unearthed was a deep commitment to that team, but perhaps different conceptions and explications and deployments of those teams over time," said Rodgers. "This is an important area of focus for us going forward." Rodgers described how the discussions then turned to the important aspects of quality, with a major focus on value. "We also highlighted the need for better payment to deliver better care," he said. In closing the workshop, Rodgers noted that despite more work to do, he is certain that with the support of the assembled community and interested organizations, progress toward further integration of serious illness care and primary care will occur.

REFERENCES

Anderson, D., V. G. Villagra, E. Coman, T. Ahmed, A. Porto, N. Jepeal, G. Maci, and B. Teevan. 2018. Reduced cost of specialty care using electronic consultations for Medicaid patients. *Health Affairs (Project Hope)* 37(12):2031–2036.

Ankuda, C. K., S. M. Petterson, O. Wingrove, and A. W. Bazemore. 2017. Regional variation primary care involvement at the end of life. *Annals of Family Medicine* 15(1):63–67.

Bailit, M. H., M. W. Friedberg, and M. L. Houy. 2017. *Standardizing the measurement of commercial health plan primary care spending*. Milbank Memorial Fund. https://www.milbank.org/publications/standardizing-measurement-commercial-health-plan-primary-care-spending (accessed September 20, 2021).

Borrell-Carrió, F., A. L. Suchman, and R. M. Epstein. 2004. The biopsychosocial model 25 years later: Principles, practice, and scientific inquiry. *The Annals of Family Medicine* 2(6):576–582.

Buttorff, C., T. Ruder, and M. Bauman. 2017. *Multiple chronic conditions in the United States*. RAND Corporation. https://www.rand.org/pubs/tools/TL221.html (accessed September 20, 2021).

CAPC (Center to Advance Palliative Care). 2021. *Patient and family resources*. https://www.capc.org/about/patient-and-family-resources (accessed November 12, 2021).

Castellucci, M. 2018. *ACEP launches accreditation program for geriatric care in emergency rooms*. Modern Healthcare. https://www.modernhealthcare.com/article/20180510/NEWS/180519985/acep-launches-accreditation-program-for-geriatric-care-in-emergency-rooms (accessed September 20, 2021).

Cornell, P. Y., C. W. Halladay, J. Ader, J. Halaszynski, M. Hogue, C. E. McClain, J. W. Silva, L. D. Taylor, and J. L. Rudolph. 2020. Embedding social workers in Veterans Health Administration primary care teams reduces emergency department visits. *Health Affairs (Millwood)* 39(4):603–612.

Edes, T. 2019. Connecting social, clinical, and home care services: Where health care needs to go. *Journal of the American Geriatric Society* 67:S419–S422.

Engel, G. L. 1977. The need for a new medical model: A challenge for biomedicine. *Science* 196:129–136.

Epstein, R. M. 1999. Mindful practice. *JAMA* 282(9):833–839.

Erickson, S. M., B. Outland, S. Joy, B. Rockwern, J. Serchen, R. D. Mire, and J. M. Goldman. 2020. Envisioning a better U.S. health care system for all: Health care delivery and payment system reforms. *Annals of Internal Medicine* 172(2 Suppl):S33–S49.

Ferrell, B. R., M. L. Twaddle, A. Melnick, and D. E. Meier. 2018. National Consensus Project clinical practice guidelines for quality palliative care guidelines, 4th edition. *Journal of Palliative Medicine* 21(12):1684–1689.

Foley, K., and C. Luz. 2021. Retooling the health care workforce for an aging America: A current perspective. *Gerontologist* 61(4):487–496.

Gallo, J. J., K. H. Morales, H. R. Bogner, P. J. Raue, J. Zee, M. L. Bruce, and C. F. Reynolds III. 2013. Long term effect of depression care management on mortality in older adults: Follow-up of cluster randomized clinical trial in primary care. *BMJ* 346:f2570.

Ghany, R., L. Tamariz, G. Chen, E. Dawkins, A. Ghany, E. Forbes, T. Tajiri, and A. Palacio. 2018. High-touch care leads to better outcomes and lower costs in a senior population. *American Journal of Managed Care* 24(9):e300–e304.

Gilbody, S., P. Bower, J. Fletcher, D. Richards, and A. J. Sutton. 2006. Collaborative care for depression: A cumulative meta-analysis and review of longer-term outcomes. *Archives of Internal Medicine* 166(21):2314–2321.

Gleason, N., P. A. Prasad, S. Ackerman, C. Ho, J. Monacelli, M. Wang, D. Collado, and R. Gonzales. 2017. Adoption and impact of an eConsult system in a fee-for-service setting. *Healthcare (Amsterdam, Netherlands)* 5(1–2):40–45.

Gorman, R. 2016. Integrating palliative care into primary care. *Nursing Clinics of North America* 51(3):367–379.

Hendricks Sloan, D., T. Peters, K. S. Johnson, J. V. Bowie, Y. Ting, and R. Aslakson. 2016. Church-based health promotion focused on advance care planning and end-of-life care at Black Baptist churches: A cross-sectional survey. *Journal of Palliative Medicine* 19(2):190–194.

Huded, J. M., A. Lee, C. M. McQuown, S. Song, M. S. Ascha, D. M. Kresevic, G. E. Maloney, and T. I. Smith. 2020. Implementation of a geriatric emergency department program using a novel workforce. *American Journal of Emergency Medicine* 46:703–707.

Hwang, U., and R. S. Morrison. 2007. The geriatric emergency department. *Journal of the American Geriatric Society* 55(11):1873–1876.

Hwang, U., S. M. Dresden, C. Vargas-Torres, R. Kang, M. M. Garrido, G. Loo, J. Sze, D. Cruz, L. D. Richardson, J. Adams, A. Aldeen, K. M. Baumlin, D. M. Courtney, S. Gravenor, C. R. Grudzen, G. Nimo, C. W. Zhu, and Geriatric Emergency Department Innovations in Care Through Workforce, Informatics and Structural Enhancement (GEDI WISE) Investigators. 2021. Association of a geriatric emergency department innovation program with cost outcomes among Medicare beneficiaries. *JAMA Network Open* 4(3):e2037334.

IOM (Institute of Medicine). 2015. *Dying in America: Improving quality and honoring individual preferences near the end of life*. Washington, DC: The National Academies Press. https://doi.org/10.17226/18748.

Kamal, A. H., M. Gradison, J. M. Maguire, D. Taylor, and A. P. Abernethy. 2014. Quality measures for palliative care in patients with cancer: A systematic review. *Journal of Oncology Practice* 10(4):281–287.

Kamal, A. H., J. M. Maguire, and D. E. Meier. 2015. Evolving the palliative care workforce to provide responsive, serious illness care. *Annals of Internal Medicine* 163(8):637–638.

Kamal, A. H., T. W. LeBlanc, and D. E. Meier. 2016. Better palliative care for all: Improving the lived experience with cancer. *JAMA* 316(1):29–30.

Kamal, A. H., S. P. Wolf, J. Troy, V. Leff, C. Dahlin, J. D. Rotella, G. Handzo, P. E. Rodgers, and E. R. Myers. 2019. Policy changes key to promoting sustainability and growth of the specialty palliative care workforce. *Health Affairs* 38(6):910–918.

Kamal, A. H., C. Bausewein, D. J. Casarett, D. C. Currow, D. J. Dudgeon, and I. J. Higginson. 2020. Standards, guidelines, and quality measures for successful specialty palliative care integration into oncology: Current approaches and future directions. *Journal of Clinical Oncology* 38(9):987–994.

Katon, W. J., E. H. B. Lin, M. Von Korff, P. Ciechanowski, E. J. Ludman, B. Young, D. Peterson, C. M. Rutter, M. McGregor, and D. McCulloch. 2010. Collaborative care for patients with depression and chronic illnesses. *The New England Journal of Medicine* 363(27):2611–2620.

Kelley, A. S., and E. Bollens-Lund. 2017. Identifying the population with serious illness: The "denominator" challenge. *Journal of Palliative Medicine* 21(S2):S-7–S-16.

Koller, C. F. 2017. *Measuring primary care health care spending*. Milbank Memorial Fund. https://www.milbank.org/2017/07/getting-primary-care-oriented-measuring-primary-care-spending (accessed September 20, 2021).

Koller, C. F., and D. Khullar. 2017. Primary care spending rate—a lever for encouraging investment in primary care. *The New England Journal of Medicine* 377(18):1709–1711.

Liddy, C., P. Drosinis, and E. Keely. 2016. Electronic consultation systems: Worldwide prevalence and their impact on patient care—a systematic review. *Family Practice* 33(3):274–285.

Loxterkamp, D. 2019. Whither family medicine? Our past, future, and enduring scope of practice. *Family Medicine* 51(7):555–558.

NASEM (National Academies of Sciences, Engineering, and Medicine). 2021. *Implementing high-quality primary care: Rebuilding the foundation of health care*. Washington, DC: The National Academies Press.

NASW (National Association of Social Workers). n.d. *Why choose the social work profession?* https://www.socialworkers.org/Careers/NASW-Career-Center/Explore-Social-Work/Why-Choose-the-Social-Work-Profession (accessed September 20, 2021).

Parikh, R., A. Lepp, and R. S. Phillips. 2015. *A more cohesive home: integrating primary and palliative care for seriously ill patients*. HealthAffairs Blog. https://www.healthaffairs.org/do/10.1377/hblog20150803.049733/full (accessed October 6, 2021).

Phillips, R. L., Jr., and A. W. Bazemore. 2010. Primary care and why it matters for U.S. health system reform. *Health Affairs (Project Hope)* 29(5):806–810.

Schmittdiel, J. A., S. M. Shortell, T. G. Rundall, T. Bodenheimer, and J. V. Selby. 2006. Effect of primary health care orientation on chronic care management. *Annals of Family Medicine* 4(2):117–123.

Starfield, B., L. Shi, and J. Macinko. 2005. Contribution of primary care to health systems and health. *Milbank Quarterly* 83(3):457–502.

Stephens, G. G. 1990. *Family practice in the 1980s: A second decade of essays*. Kansas City, MO: Society of Teachers of Family Medicine Foundation.

Tinetti, M. E., D. M. Costello, A. D. Naik, C. Davenport, K. Hernandez-Bigos, J. R. Van Liew, J. Esterson, E. Kiwak, and L. Dindo. 2021. Outcome goals and health care preferences of older adults with multiple chronic conditions. *JAMA Network Open* 4(3):e211271.

Unützer, J., W. Katon, C. M. Callahan, J. W. Williams, Jr., E. Hunkeler, L. Haropole, M. Hoffing, R. D. Della Penna, P. Hitchcock Noel, E. H. B. Lin, P. A. Arean, M. T. Hegel, L. Tang, T. R. Belin, S. Oishi, and C. Langston. 2002. Collaborative care management of late-life depression in the primary care setting: A randomized controlled trial. *JAMA* 288(22):2836–2845.

Vimalananda, V. G., G. Gupte, S. M. Seraj, J. Orlander, D. Berlowitz, B. G. Fincke, and S. R. Simon. 2015. Electronic consultations (e-consults) to improve access to specialty care: A systematic review and narrative synthesis. *Journal of Telemedicine and Telecare* 21(6):323–330.

White, N., N. Kupeli, V. Vickerstaff, and P. Stone. 2017. How accurate is the "Surprise Question" at identifying patients at the end of life? A systematic review and meta-analysis. *BMC Medicine* 15(1):139.

A

Statement of Task

A planning committee of the National Academies of Sciences, Engineering, and Medicine will organize and host a 1-day workshop to examine approaches to improving the ability of primary care clinicians to care for people with serious illness across care settings, with an emphasis on palliative care principles, practices, policies, and payment mechanisms.

The workshop will feature invited presentations and panel discussions on topics that may include:

- The central role of primary care in providing high-quality care for people with serious illness;
- Changing patient demographics and workforce needs;
- Education and training challenges and opportunities to develop serious illness care; competencies for interdisciplinary primary care clinicians that are informed by principles and practices of high-quality palliative care;
- Barriers, facilitators, and effective models of care delivery for integrating serious illness care delivery into primary care settings;
- Impact of integrating serious illness care into primary care delivery on patient satisfaction, quality of care, and cost of care;
- Regulatory and payment policy mechanisms to support integrating serious illness care into primary care practices; and

- Key areas for further research to advance serious illness care integration in primary care settings.

The planning committee will develop the agenda for the workshop, select speakers and discussants, and moderate the discussions. A proceedings of the presentations and discussions at the workshop will be prepared by a designated rapporteur in accordance with institutional guidelines.

B

Workshop Agenda

WEBINAR 1: JUNE 10, 2021
12:00–3:00 PM ET

12:00 PM   **Welcome from the Roundtable on Quality Care for People with Serious Illness**

                 Peggy Maguire, J.D.
                 Cambia Health Foundation

                 James Tulsky, M.D.
                 Dana-Farber Cancer Institute, Brigham and Women's Hospital, Harvard Medical School

                 Roundtable Co-Chairs

12:05 PM   **Overview of the Virtual Workshop**

                 Patricia Davidson, Ph.D.
                 Vice Chancellor, University of Wollongong, Australia (*as of April 2021*)
                 Dean, Johns Hopkins University School of Nursing (*through March 2021*)

Phillip Rodgers, M.D., FAAHPM
Professor, Family Medicine and Internal Medicine
Co-Director, Clinical Palliative Care Program
University of Michigan School of Medicine

Planning Committee Co-Chairs

12:10 PM SESSION ONE: Exploring the Shared Principles of Serious Illness Care and Primary Care

Opening Remarks:
Ada D. Stewart, M.D., FAAFP
President
American Academy of Family Physicians

Claire Ankuda, M.D., M.P.H.
Assistant Professor, Geriatrics and Palliative Medicine
Icahn School of Medicine at Mount Sinai

Speakers:
Shirley Roberson
C-TAC Fellow
Member, Board of Directors

Erin Bradshaw
Chief of Mission Delivery
Patient Advocate Foundation

Martha L. Twaddle, M.D.
Waud Family Medical Director for Palliative Medicine & Supportive Care
Northwestern's North Region
Clinical Professor of Medicine, Northwestern University Feinberg School of Medicine

Carlos Roberto Jaén, M.D., Ph.D., M.S., FAAFP
Dr. and Mrs. James L. Holly Distinguished Chair, Patient-Centered Medical Home, and Professor and Chair of Family and Community Medicine and Professor of Population Health Sciences
Joe R. and Teresa Lozano Long School of Medicine, University of Texas Health San Antonio
Adjunct Professor of Public Health, University of Texas Health School of Public Health

12:50 PM Panel Discussion

1:15 PM Audience Q&A

1:30 PM **SESSION TWO: The Role of Interdisciplinary Teams in Caring for People with Serious Illness in Primary Care Settings**

Moderator:
Lori Bishop M.H.A., B.S.N., RN
Vice President of Palliative and Advanced Care
National Hospice and Palliative Care Organization

Speakers:
Marianne Logan Fingerhood, DNP, CRNP, ANP-BC
Track Coordinator Adult/Gerontological NP Program
Supporting Nursing Advanced Practice Transitions Nurse Practitioner Fellowship Program Director
Assistant Professor, Johns Hopkins University School of Nursing

Karen Bullock, Ph.D.
Professor and Head of the School of Social Work
North Carolina State University

Gregg VandeKieft, M.D., M.A., FAAFP, FAAHPM
Medical Director, Palliative Practice Group
Providence Institute for Human Caring
Palliative Care Physician, Clinical Ethicist
Providence St. Peter Hospital

Danetta E. Sloan, Ph.D., M.S.W., M.A.
Assistant Scientist
Johns Hopkins Bloomberg School of Public Health

Russell S. Phillips, M.D.
Director, Center for Primary Care
Harvard Medical School

2:25 PM   Panel Discussion

2:45 PM   Audience Q&A

3:00 PM   Closing Remarks/Webinar Adjourns

WEBINAR 2: JUNE 17, 2021
12:00–3:00 PM ET

12:00 PM   Welcome from the Roundtable on Quality Care for People with Serious Illness

Peggy Maguire, J.D.
Cambia Health Foundation

James Tulsky, M.D.
Dana-Farber Cancer Institute, Brigham and Women's Hospital, Harvard Medical School

Roundtable Co-Chairs

Patricia Davidson, Ph.D.
Vice Chancellor, University of Wollongong, Australia
(*as of April 2021*)
Dean, Johns Hopkins University School of Nursing
(*through March 2021*)

APPENDIX B

Phillip Rodgers, M.D., FAAHPM
Professor, Family Medicine and Internal Medicine
Co-Director, Clinical Palliative Care Program
University of Michigan School of Medicine

Planning Committee Co-Chairs

12:05 PM **Opening Remarks**

Brief Summary of the First Webinar:
Patricia Davidson, Ph.D.

Patient Voice:
Mike Olex
Volunteer, National Patient Advocate Foundation

12:20 PM **SESSION THREE: Policy Mechanisms to Support Person-Centered Care for People with Serious Illness in Primary Care Settings**

Moderator:
Phil Rodgers, M.D.

Speakers:
Arif Kamal M.D., M.B.A., M.H.S.
Associate Professor of Medicine
Duke University

Amy Bassano, M.A.
Deputy Director, Center for Medicare & Medicaid Innovation
Centers for Medicare & Medicaid Services

Megan Thompson, M.A.
Senior Policy Advisor
Office of Senator Jacky Rosen (D-NV)
U.S. Senate

Kimberly Bower, M.D., FAAHPM, HMDC
Medical Director
Blue Shield of California Promise Health Plan

Adam M. Barde, M.H.A., M.S.G.
Senior Director, Health Transformation Implementation
Health Transformation & Network Development
Blue Shield of California

1:05 PM   **Panel Discussion**

1:25 PM   **Audience Q&A**

1:40 PM   **SESSION FOUR: Promising Integrated Care Models**

Moderator:
Lars Peterson, M.D., Ph.D.
Vice President of Research
American Board of Family Medicine

Speakers:
Deborah M. Swiderski, M.D.
Associate Professor of Medicine and Family and Social
   Medicine
Albert Einstein College of Medicine
Montefiore Medical Center

Faisel Syed, M.D.
National Director for Primary Care
ChenMed

Thomas E. Edes, M.D., M.S.
Senior Medical Advisor
Geriatrics & Extended Care
U.S. Department of Veterans Affairs

Neela K. Patel, M.D., M.P.H., CMD
Associate Professor, Joe R. and Teresa Lozano Long Chair in
  Geriatrics and Senior Care
Chief, Division of Geriatrics and Palliative Care
Departments of Family and Community Medicine
University of Texas Health San Antonio

2:20 PM **Panel Discussion**

2:40 PM **Audience Q&A**

2:55 PM **Closing Remarks/Wrap-Up for the Virtual Workshop**

3:00 PM **Webinar Adjourns**